"Fundamentals of Diabetic Cooking: A Beginner's Guide"

"Dive into the world of diabetic cooking with confidence and ease through 'Fundamentals of Diabetic Cooking: A Beginner's Guide.' This comprehensive manual equips you with essential knowledge, practical tips, and delectable recipes tailored specifically for beginners navigating the realm of diabetic-friendly cuisine. Discover how to create flavorful meals that not only support your health but also delight your taste buds. With step-by-step guidance and insightful advice, embark on a journey toward mastering the art of diabetic cooking and embrace a lifestyle filled with delicious, wholesome meals."

index:

1. Introduction

   - Understanding Diabetes

   - Importance of Diet in Diabetes Management

   - Tips for Cooking with Diabetes

2. Breakfast Recipes

   - Healthy Oatmeal Varieties

   - Low-Carb Breakfast Casseroles

   - Sugar-Free Smoothie Creations

3. Lunch Ideas

   - Balanced Salad Options

Chapter 1

"Introduction"

Introduction

Welcome to "The Complete Diabetic Cookbook for Beginners," where we embark on a journey of culinary exploration and empowerment in the realm of diabetes management. In this comprehensive guide, we delve into the multifaceted dimensions of living and thriving with diabetes, from understanding the intricacies of this metabolic disorder to harnessing the power of nutrition and cooking to optimize health and well-being.

As we navigate the pages of this cookbook, we invite you to embrace cooking not merely as a means of sustenance but as a form of self-expression, creativity, and self-care. Through mindful ingredient selection, culinary experimentation, and flavor exploration, we aim to transform your kitchen into a sanctuary of health, flavor, and empowerment.

With each recipe, tip, and strategy shared within these pages, our goal is to equip you with the knowledge, skills, and confidence to navigate the culinary landscape with diabetes with ease and joy. Whether you're a seasoned home cook or just beginning your culinary journey, this cookbook is designed to inspire and empower you to discover the joys of delicious, diabetes-friendly cooking.

1.1. Understanding Diabetes

Understanding diabetes goes beyond recognizing it as a medical condition characterized by high blood sugar levels. It delves into the intricate web of physiological processes, lifestyle implications, and emotional impacts that encompass the diabetic journey. At its core, comprehending diabetes is about embracing a holistic perspective that empowers individuals to navigate their health with knowledge, resilience, and compassion.

The Physiology of Diabetes

Diabetes is a metabolic disorder rooted in the body's inability to produce or effectively utilize insulin, a hormone crucial for regulating blood sugar levels. In type 1 diabetes, the immune system mistakenly attacks and destroys insulin-producing beta cells in the pancreas, leading to insulin deficiency. On the other hand, type 2 diabetes typically arises from a combination of insulin resistance, where cells fail to respond adequately to insulin, and pancreatic beta cell dysfunction.

Beyond its immediate impact on blood sugar regulation, diabetes affects various organ systems, including the cardiovascular, nervous, and renal systems. Chronic hyperglycemia, or consistently elevated blood sugar levels, can contribute to a cascade of complications such as cardiovascular disease, neuropathy, nephropathy, and retinopathy. Understanding these interconnected physiological pathways underscores the importance of proactive diabetes management to mitigate long-term complications.

The Spectrum of Diabetes

Diabetes is not a one-size-fits-all condition, but rather exists along a spectrum, encompassing diverse manifestations and individual experiences. While type 1 and type 2 diabetes represent the most prevalent forms, gestational diabetes, prediabetes, and monogenic diabetes add layers of complexity to the diagnostic landscape. Each subtype carries distinct genetic, environmental, and lifestyle factors that influence its onset, progression, and management.

Moreover, diabetes intersects with various other health conditions, such as obesity, hypertension, and dyslipidemia, forming intricate comorbidities that demand personalized care approaches. Recognizing the multifaceted nature of diabetes fosters empathy, solidarity, and inclusivity within the diabetic community, acknowledging that no two journeys are identical.

Lifestyle and Behavioral Considerations

Beyond its physiological underpinnings, diabetes permeates every aspect of daily life, shaping choices related to diet, exercise, medication adherence, and emotional well-being. Dietary habits play a pivotal role in glycemic control, with carbohydrate counting, portion control, and glycemic index awareness serving as foundational principles. Physical activity acts synergistically with insulin sensitivity, promoting glucose uptake by muscles and enhancing overall metabolic health.

Moreover, the emotional toll of living with diabetes cannot be overstated, as individuals navigate feelings of frustration, fear, and stigma amidst their health journey. Understanding the psychosocial dimensions of diabetes entails fostering open dialogue, cultivating resilience, and destigmatizing misconceptions surrounding the condition.

Empowerment Through Education

Central to understanding diabetes is the empowerment derived from education, advocacy, and self-advocacy. Equipping individuals with comprehensive knowledge about their condition instills confidence, autonomy, and agency in managing their health effectively. From deciphering blood glucose readings to mastering insulin administration techniques, education serves as a cornerstone for fostering diabetes self-management skills.

Furthermore, advocating for equitable access to healthcare resources, diabetes education programs, and supportive communities is essential for dismantling barriers to optimal diabetes care. By amplifying diverse voices, challenging societal norms, and fostering inclusivity, we can cultivate a more compassionate and supportive ecosystem for individuals living with diabetes.

In essence, understanding diabetes transcends mere medical knowledge; it embodies a profound journey of self-discovery, resilience, and community. By embracing a holistic perspective that integrates physiological insights with lifestyle considerations and empowering individuals through education and advocacy, we can foster a brighter future where diabetes is not just managed but lived with vitality and purpose.

1.2. Importance of Diet in Diabetes Management

Dietary choices wield unparalleled influence in the realm of diabetes management, serving as a cornerstone for achieving optimal blood sugar control, preventing complications, and fostering overall well-being. The significance of diet extends far beyond mere sustenance; it embodies a powerful tool for empowering individuals to take charge of their health, nourish their bodies, and thrive in the face of diabetes.

Balancing Macronutrients

At the heart of diabetes management lies the delicate balance of macronutrients—carbohydrates, proteins, and fats. Carbohydrates, in particular, hold a central role due to their direct impact on blood glucose levels. By understanding the glycemic index and glycemic load of various carbohydrate sources, individuals can make informed choices that promote steady blood sugar levels and minimize postprandial spikes.

Proteins play a crucial role in muscle repair, satiety, and metabolic function, making them an essential component of a balanced diabetic diet. Incorporating lean protein sources such as poultry, fish, tofu, and legumes not only supports blood sugar control but also aids in weight management and muscle preservation.

Similarly, dietary fats, when consumed in moderation and from healthy sources such as avocados, nuts, seeds, and olive oil, contribute to satiety, hormone regulation, and cardiovascular health. Embracing a balanced approach to macronutrient intake ensures sustained energy levels, promotes satiety, and optimizes metabolic function in individuals living with diabetes.

Navigating Carbohydrates Wisely

Carbohydrate management lies at the crux of diabetes dietary guidelines, as these macronutrients exert the most significant impact on blood sugar levels. However, rather than adopting a blanket approach to carb restriction, the focus shifts towards quality and portion control. Whole grains, fruits, vegetables, and legumes offer nutrient-dense sources of carbohydrates rich in fiber, vitamins, and minerals, promoting satiety and stabilizing blood sugar levels.

Portion control emerges as a pivotal strategy for managing carbohydrate intake, allowing individuals to enjoy their favorite foods while maintaining glycemic control. Tools such as carbohydrate counting, plate method visualization, and glycemic index awareness empower individuals to make mindful choices that align with their dietary preferences and metabolic needs.

Moreover, the concept of carbohydrate consistency underscores the importance of distributing carbohydrate intake evenly throughout the day, thereby preventing blood sugar fluctuations and optimizing insulin sensitivity. By incorporating slow-digesting carbohydrates, such as whole grains and fibrous vegetables, into meals and snacks, individuals can achieve sustained energy levels and avoid the peaks and valleys associated with rapid glucose spikes.

Embracing Nutrient-Dense Foods

Beyond macronutrient composition, the focus shifts towards embracing a diet rich in nutrient-dense foods that nourish the body and support overall health. Fresh fruits and vegetables, brimming with vitamins, minerals, and antioxidants, form the foundation of a diabetes-friendly diet, offering an array of flavors, textures, and culinary possibilities.

Lean protein sources, such as poultry, fish, eggs, and plant-based alternatives, provide essential amino acids for muscle repair and metabolic function, while also promoting satiety and aiding in weight management. Incorporating healthy fats from sources like avocados, nuts, seeds, and olive oil enhances flavor, texture, and satiety without compromising metabolic health.

Moreover, prioritizing whole, minimally processed foods over their refined counterparts allows individuals to reap the full spectrum of nutrients while minimizing exposure to added sugars, sodium, and preservatives. By fostering a culture of culinary creativity, experimentation, and enjoyment, individuals can transform their dietary habits into a source of empowerment, pleasure, and vitality.

Cultivating Mindful Eating Practices

In the bustling landscape of modern-day living, cultivating mindful eating practices emerges as a transformative strategy for enhancing dietary awareness, savoring the sensory experience of food, and fostering a deeper connection with one's body. Mindful eating encompasses a spectrum of practices, from savoring each bite and tuning into hunger and satiety cues, to practicing gratitude for the nourishment provided by food.

By slowing down the pace of eating, minimizing distractions, and savoring the flavors, textures, and aromas of food, individuals can enhance their satisfaction, promote digestion, and prevent overeating. Moreover, mindful eating cultivates a non-judgmental awareness of food choices, allowing individuals to navigate cravings, emotional eating triggers, and social influences with greater resilience and self-compassion.

In essence, the importance of diet in diabetes management transcends mere caloric intake; it embodies a dynamic interplay of macronutrient balance, carbohydrate awareness, nutrient density, and mindful eating practices. By embracing a holistic approach that celebrates the diversity and vibrancy of whole foods, individuals can harness the power of nutrition to thrive in their diabetic journey, nourishing their bodies, minds, and spirits with intention and vitality.

1.3. Tips for Cooking with Diabetes

Navigating the culinary landscape with diabetes requires a blend of creativity, mindfulness, and culinary know-how. By embracing cooking as a form of self-expression and self-care, individuals can transform their kitchen into a sanctuary of health, flavor, and empowerment. Here, we explore practical tips and strategies for cooking with diabetes, from ingredient selection and cooking techniques to meal planning and flavor enhancement.

Embracing Flavorful, Nutrient-Dense Ingredients

At the heart of diabetes-friendly cooking lies the art of ingredient selection, where fresh, whole foods take center stage as the building blocks of delicious, nourishing meals. Fruits and vegetables, bursting with vibrant colors, flavors, and nutrients, form the foundation of a balanced diabetic diet, offering an array of culinary possibilities. Opt for seasonal produce to maximize flavor and nutritional value while supporting local farmers and reducing environmental impact.

Whole grains, such as quinoa, brown rice, and barley, serve as wholesome alternatives to refined grains, providing fiber, vitamins, and minerals that promote satiety and stabilize blood sugar levels. Incorporating lean protein sources, including poultry, fish, tofu, and legumes, adds depth and richness to dishes while supporting muscle repair and metabolic function.

Moreover, don't shy away from incorporating healthy fats from sources like avocados, nuts, seeds, and olive oil, which enhance flavor, texture, and satiety without compromising metabolic health. By embracing a diverse array of nutrient-dense ingredients, individuals can elevate their culinary creations while nourishing their bodies and supporting optimal health.

Mastering Cooking Techniques for Diabetes-Friendly Meals

Cooking with diabetes invites exploration and experimentation with a variety of cooking techniques that enhance flavor, texture, and nutritional value without relying on excessive fats, sugars, or salt. Embrace methods such as roasting, grilling, steaming, and sautéing to coax out the natural flavors of ingredients while preserving their integrity and nutritional content.

For example, roasting vegetables at high heat caramelizes their natural sugars, resulting in tender, flavorful morsels that require minimal seasoning. Similarly, grilling imparts a smoky depth to proteins and vegetables, lending a tantalizing charred aroma and flavor that enhances the dining experience.

Steaming preserves the delicate textures and vibrant colors of vegetables while minimizing nutrient loss, making it an ideal technique for preserving their nutritional integrity. Sautéing, with a modest amount of heart-healthy olive oil, allows for quick cooking while imparting rich, savory flavors to dishes.

Mindful Meal Planning and Portion Control

Effective meal planning lies at the core of successful diabetes management, offering structure, consistency, and balance to daily eating habits. Begin by mapping out a weekly menu that incorporates a variety of nutrient-dense foods, including lean proteins, whole grains, fruits, and vegetables, to ensure a diverse array of flavors and nutrients.Consider portion control as a key component of meal planning, aiming to fill half of your plate with non-starchy vegetables, one-quarter with lean protein, and one-quarter with whole grains or starchy vegetables. Use smaller plates and bowls to visually cue appropriate portion sizes and prevent overeating, and consider pre-portioning snacks and leftovers to promote mindful eating habits.

Enhancing Flavor Without Compromise

Flavor enhancement in diabetes-friendly cooking revolves around harnessing the natural aromas, textures, and tastes of ingredients through mindful seasoning and flavor pairing. Experiment with herbs, spices, citrus zest, and vinegars to add depth, complexity, and brightness to dishes without relying on excessive salt or sugar.

For example, a sprinkle of fresh herbs such as basil, cilantro, or parsley can elevate the flavor profile of a simple salad or grilled fish. Likewise, spices such as cinnamon, cumin, and turmeric offer warm, earthy notes that complement a variety of savory and sweet dishes while providing antioxidant and anti-inflammatory benefits.

Explore the nuanced flavors of different vinegar varieties, from balsamic and red wine vinegar to apple cider and rice vinegar, to add acidity and brightness to dressings, marinades, and sauces. By embracing a culinary palette rich in diverse flavors and textures, individuals can savor the joys of cooking while supporting their health and well-being.

In essence, cooking with diabetes transcends mere sustenance; it embodies a journey of creativity, mindfulness, and culinary exploration. By embracing fresh, nutrient-dense ingredients, mastering cooking techniques that enhance flavor and nutritional value, and practicing mindful meal planning and portion control, individuals can transform their kitchen into a sanctuary of health, flavor, and empowerment.

Conclusion

As we conclude our exploration of the introduction to "The Complete Diabetic Cookbook for Beginners," we're reminded of the transformative power of food and cooking in the realm of diabetes management. Through understanding the physiology of diabetes, embracing the importance of a balanced diet, and mastering cooking techniques tailored to diabetes-friendly meals, we've laid the groundwork for a journey of culinary empowerment and well-being.

In the bustling landscape of modern-day living, where convenience often trumps conscientiousness, it's easy to overlook the profound impact that food choices can have on our health and vitality. Yet, as we've discovered, by embracing fresh, whole ingredients, mindful cooking techniques, and flavor enhancement strategies, we can unlock the full potential of nutrition as a tool for optimizing health and managing diabetes with confidence and joy.

As you embark on your culinary journey with "The Complete Diabetic Cookbook for Beginners," we encourage you to approach cooking not as a chore but as a source of pleasure, creativity, and self-discovery. With each meal prepared with love and intention, may you nourish not only your body but also your spirit, embracing the joys of delicious, diabetes-friendly cooking as a pathway to vibrant health and well-being.

Chapter 2

"Breakfast Recipes"

Introduction

Welcome to the tantalizing world of breakfast recipes, where creativity, flavor, and nourishment converge to kicks tart your day on a delicious note. In this chapter, we embark on a culinary journey through a diverse array of morning delights, from hearty oatmeal varieties and low-carb breakfast casseroles to refreshing sugar-free smoothie creations. Whether you're seeking a comforting bowl of oats to fuel your morning or a protein-packed smoothie to invigorate your senses, this chapter is your guide to crafting nutritious and satisfying breakfast options that cater to a variety of tastes and dietary preferences.

As we delve into the recipes and techniques shared within these pages, we invite you to embrace breakfast not merely as a meal but as a moment of nourishment, pleasure, and self-care. From the comforting aroma of freshly cooked oats to the vibrant colors of a blended smoothie, each recipe serves as an invitation to savor the simple joys of starting your day with intention and vitality. Whether you're cooking for yourself, your family, or guests, let these breakfast recipes inspire you to elevate your morning routine with delicious, diabetes-friendly options that nourish the body and delight the senses.

2.1. Healthy Oatmeal Varieties

Oatmeal stands as a quintessential breakfast option, cherished for its versatility, simplicity, and nutritional prowess. Beyond its humble appearance, oatmeal serves as a canvas for culinary creativity, offering a myriad of healthy variations to suit every palate and dietary preference. In this exploration of healthy oatmeal varieties, we uncover the diverse array of flavors, textures, and toppings that elevate this breakfast staple from mundane to magnificent.

Classic Rolled Oats

At the heart of healthy oatmeal varieties lies the classic rolled oats, prized for their hearty texture and nutty flavor profile. Rolled oats, also known as old-fashioned oats, undergo minimal processing, retaining their natural bran and germ layers rich in fiber, vitamins, and minerals. To prepare classic rolled oats, simply simmer them in water or milk until creamy and tender, stirring occasionally to prevent sticking.

Steel-Cut Oats

For those seeking a heartier, chewier oatmeal experience, steel-cut oats offer a delightful alternative. Made by slicing whole oat groats into smaller pieces, steel-cut oats boast a robust texture and nutty flavor that pairs beautifully with a variety of toppings. While steel-cut oats require a longer cooking time compared to rolled oats, their satisfying bite and nutritional density make them worth the extra effort.

Overnight Oats

In today's fast-paced world, convenience reigns supreme, making overnight oats a popular choice for busy mornings. This no-cook oatmeal variation involves soaking oats in liquid—such as milk, yogurt, or plant-based alternatives—overnight in the refrigerator, allowing them to soften and absorb the flavors of added ingredients. From chia seeds and fresh fruit to nut butter and spices, the customization options for overnight oats are endless, offering a convenient and nutritious breakfast solution for hectic schedules.

Savory Oatmeal Bowls

While oatmeal is often associated with sweet toppings such as fruit, nuts, and honey, savory oatmeal bowls offer a savory twist that tantalizes the taste buds and satisfies hunger cravings. Start with a base of cooked oats and incorporate savory ingredients such as sautéed vegetables, poached eggs, avocado slices, and grated cheese. Experiment with flavor combinations inspired by global cuisines, such as Mediterranean-inspired toppings with olives, tomatoes, and feta cheese, or Mexican-inspired toppings with salsa, black beans, and cilantro.

Protein-Packed Oatmeal

For individuals seeking to boost their protein intake at breakfast, protein-packed oatmeal varieties offer a satisfying solution. Incorporate protein-rich ingredients such as Greek yogurt, cottage cheese, protein powder, or nut butter into your oatmeal base to add creaminess, flavor, and satiety. Top with additional protein sources such as chopped nuts, seeds, or hemp hearts for an extra nutritional boost that fuels you through the morning.

Toppings and Garnishes

The beauty of oatmeal lies in its adaptability to a wide range of toppings and garnishes that cater to individual tastes and preferences. From fresh fruit and dried berries to nuts, seeds, and spices, the possibilities for oatmeal toppings are limited only by imagination. Experiment with seasonal ingredients, flavor combinations, and textures to create customized oatmeal bowls that delight the senses and nourish the body.

Conclusion

In conclusion, healthy oatmeal varieties offer a delicious and nutritious breakfast option that caters to a diverse range of tastes, preferences, and dietary needs. Whether you prefer classic rolled oats, hearty steel-cut oats, or convenient overnight oats, there's a perfect oatmeal variation to suit every palate and lifestyle. By exploring savory oatmeal bowls, protein-packed options, and a myriad of creative toppings and garnishes, individuals can elevate their morning routine with a satisfying and nourishing meal that sets the tone for a productive and energized day ahead.

2.2. Low-Carb Breakfast Casseroles

In the realm of breakfast cuisine, casseroles stand as a beloved and versatile option, offering a convenient way to prepare hearty, satisfying meals ahead of time. For individuals following a low-carb lifestyle, breakfast casseroles present an opportunity to indulge in flavorful creations without compromising their dietary goals. In this exploration of low-carb breakfast casseroles, we delve into innovative recipes, creative ingredient substitutions, and cooking tips to elevate your morning routine with delicious, diabetes-friendly options.

Choosing Low-Carb Ingredients

The key to crafting low-carb breakfast casseroles lies in selecting ingredients that are naturally low in carbohydrates while rich in flavor, texture, and nutritional value. Opt for protein-rich ingredients such as eggs, lean meats, poultry, and seafood as the base of your casserole, providing essential amino acids for muscle repair and satiety.

Incorporate an array of non-starchy vegetables such as spinach, bell peppers, mushrooms, and broccoli to add bulk, fiber, and micronutrients to your casserole while keeping carbohydrate content in check. Experiment with flavor-enhancing ingredients such as onions, garlic, herbs, and spices to elevate the taste profile of your dish without relying on added sugars or high-carb condiments.

Egg-Based Casseroles

Eggs serve as a versatile and nutritious foundation for low-carb breakfast casseroles, offering a rich source of protein, vitamins, and minerals with minimal carbohydrates. Whip up a classic frittata or crustless quiche using a combination of eggs, vegetables, and cheese for a satisfying meal that's both hearty and low in carbs.

For added variety, explore international flavors by incorporating ingredients inspired by cuisines from around the world. For example, create a Mediterranean-inspired frittata with spinach, feta cheese, sun-dried tomatoes, and olives, or a Tex-Mex quiche with diced green chilies, shredded chicken, and pepper jack cheese.

Vegetable-Forward Creations

Vegetable-forward casseroles offer a delicious and nutritious way to boost your vegetable intake while keeping carbohydrates in check. Layer thinly sliced vegetables such as zucchini, eggplant, and yellow squash to create a colorful and flavorful base for your casserole.

For added protein and flavor, incorporate plant-based ingredients such as tofu, tempeh, or legumes into your casserole mixture. Experiment with different seasoning blends and sauces to enhance the taste profile of your dish, from Italian-inspired marinara sauce to Asian-inspired soy ginger glaze.

Crestless Quiches and Breakfast Bakes

Crestless quiches and breakfast bakes serve as convenient and customizable options for low-carb breakfast casseroles. Simply combine eggs, milk or non-dairy alternatives, and your choice of fillings such as vegetables, cheese, and cooked meats in a baking dish, then bake until set and golden brown.

Experiment with different flavor combinations to suit your taste preferences and dietary needs, from classic combinations like ham and cheese to more adventurous options like spinach and feta or mushroom and Swiss. Serve your crustless quiche or breakfast bake hot out of the oven for a satisfying and nutritious start to your day.

Make-Ahead Convenience

One of the greatest advantages of low-carb breakfast casseroles is their make-ahead convenience, allowing you to prepare a batch of delicious, diabetes-friendly meals in advance and enjoy them throughout the week. Simply assemble your casserole, cover and refrigerate or freeze until ready to bake, then reheat individual servings as needed for a quick and satisfying breakfast on the go.

By incorporating low-carb ingredients, exploring innovative recipes, and embracing make-ahead convenience, you can elevate your morning routine with delicious and nutritious low-carb breakfast casseroles that support your health and well-being. Whether you prefer egg-based creations, vegetable-forward dishes, or crustless quiches and breakfast bakes, there's a low-carb casserole option to suit every taste and lifestyle.

2.3. Sugar-Free Smoothie Creations

Smoothies stand as a refreshing and nutritious option for breakfast, offering a convenient way to pack a plethora of vitamins, minerals, and antioxidants into a single glass. For individuals seeking to minimize their sugar intake while still indulging in the delights of a morning smoothie, sugar-free creations present an opportunity to enjoy vibrant flavors and nourishing ingredients without the added sweetness. In this exploration of sugar-free smoothie creations, we unveil a medley of inventive recipes, flavor combinations, and ingredient substitutions to elevate your morning routine with delicious, diabetes-friendly options.

Base Ingredients for Sugar-Free Smoothies

The foundation of any sugar-free smoothie lies in selecting the right combination of base ingredients to create a creamy, satisfying texture without relying on added sugars or high-carb fruits. Opt for low-sugar or sugar-free alternatives such as unsweetened almond milk, coconut milk, or Greek yogurt to provide creaminess and richness to your smoothie without spiking blood sugar levels.

Incorporate nutrient-dense ingredients such as leafy greens, avocado, and cauliflower to add fiber, vitamins, and minerals to your smoothie while keeping carbohydrates in check. These ingredients not only contribute to a thick and creamy texture but also impart a subtle sweetness and earthy flavor that pairs well with a variety of fruits and flavorings.

Low-Glycemic Fruits and Flavor Enhancers

While many traditional smoothie recipes rely on high-sugar fruits such as bananas, mangoes, and pineapple for sweetness, sugar-free smoothie creations embrace low-glycemic alternatives that provide sweetness without causing rapid blood sugar spikes. Choose fruits such as berries, cherries, apples, and pears, which boast a lower sugar content and a wealth of antioxidants, vitamins, and fiber.Experiment with flavor enhancers such as cinnamon, vanilla extract, ginger, and unsweetened cocoa powder to add depth, complexity, and warmth to your smoothie without relying on added sugars. These aromatic spices and extracts not only enhance the taste profile of your smoothie but also offer a host of health benefits, from regulating blood sugar levels to supporting digestion and immune function.

Protein-Packed Smoothie Boosters

To create a balanced and satisfying sugar-free smoothie, consider incorporating protein-packed ingredients that promote satiety, muscle repair, and metabolic function. Add a scoop of high-quality protein powder—such as whey, pea, or collagen—to your smoothie to boost its protein content without adding unnecessary sugars or carbohydrates.

Alternatively, incorporate protein-rich foods such as silken tofu, Greek yogurt, cottage cheese, or nut butter into your smoothie to provide creaminess, thickness, and a satisfying texture. These ingredients not only enhance the nutritional profile of your smoothie but also contribute to long-lasting energy and satiety throughout the morning.

Fiber-Rich Additions and Superfood Superstars

To further enhance the nutritional value of your sugar-free smoothie, consider incorporating fiber-rich additions and superfood superstars that offer a wealth of health benefits. Add a handful of spinach, kale, or Swiss chard to your smoothie to boost its fiber content and add a vibrant green hue without altering the flavor profile.

Experiment with nutrient-dense superfoods such as chia seeds, flaxseeds, hemp hearts, and spirulina to add a nutritional boost to your smoothie while enhancing its texture and thickness. These superfood additions not only provide essential fatty acids, amino acids, and antioxidants but also contribute to a feeling of fullness and satisfaction.

Customization and Creative Flavor Combinations

The beauty of sugar-free smoothie creations lies in their versatility and adaptability to suit individual tastes, preferences, and dietary needs. Experiment with different flavor combinations by combining fruits, vegetables, spices, and flavorings to create unique and delicious smoothie creations that tantalize the taste buds and nourish the body.

From classic combinations such as berry-banana or tropical mango-pineapple to more adventurous options like ginger-peach or spinach-kiwi, the possibilities for sugar-free smoothie creations are limited only by imagination. Customize your smoothie to suit your nutritional goals and flavor preferences, whether you prefer a refreshing fruit smoothie, a creamy green smoothie, or a decadent chocolate smoothie.

Conclusion

In conclusion, sugar-free smoothie creations offer a delicious and nutritious way to start your day on a refreshing and energizing note without the added sugars or high-carb fruits found in traditional smoothie recipes. By selecting low-glycemic fruits, flavor enhancers, protein-packed boosters, and fiber-rich additions, you can create a balanced and satisfying smoothie that supports your health and well-being while tantalizing your taste buds. With a plethora of ingredients, flavor combinations, and customization options at your disposal, sugar-free smoothie creations invite you to embark on a culinary adventure that celebrates the vibrant flavors and nourishing benefits of whole foods. Whether you prefer a fruity concoction, a creamy green blend, or a decadent chocolate treat, there's a sugar-free smoothie creation to suit every palate and lifestyle, making it easy and enjoyable to incorporate nutritious, diabetes-friendly options into your morning routine.

Conclusion

As we conclude our exploration of breakfast recipes, we're reminded of the transformative power of food to nourish, energize, and uplift both body and spirit. From the hearty comfort of oatmeal varieties to the savory delights of low-carb breakfast casseroles and the refreshing simplicity of sugar-free smoothie creations, each recipe offers a unique opportunity to embrace the joys of cooking and eating with intention.

As you incorporate these breakfast recipes into your culinary repertoire, may you discover the pleasure of starting your day with nourishing meals that support your health and well-being. Whether you prefer the warmth of a comforting bowl of oatmeal on a chilly morning or the refreshing vitality of a vibrant smoothie on a hot day, may each bite and sip remind you of the abundance of flavors, textures, and possibilities that await in the kitchen. With each recipe shared within these pages, we invite you to infuse your morning routine with creativity, mindfulness, and joy, savoring the simple pleasures of delicious, diabetes-friendly breakfast options that nourish your body, awaken your senses, and set the stage for a day filled with vitality and well-being.

Chapter 3

"Lunch Ideas"

Introduction

Welcome to the vibrant and flavorful world of lunch ideas designed with diabetes management in mind. In this chapter, we explore a diverse array of lunch options that prioritize balanced nutrition, delicious flavors, and convenience for individuals living with diabetes. From hearty salads and flavorful soups to satisfying wraps and sandwiches, these lunch ideas are crafted to nourish the body, satisfy hunger, and support overall well-being.

Our aim is to provide inspiration and guidance for creating meals that not only meet the dietary needs of individuals with diabetes but also excite the taste buds and ignite a passion for healthy eating. With a focus on wholesome ingredients, creative flavor combinations, and mindful portion sizes, these lunch ideas offer a delicious and satisfying way to fuel your day while managing blood sugar levels and promoting optimal health.

Whether you're preparing lunch for yourself, your family, or guests, we invite you to explore the possibilities and embrace the joy of cooking and eating with intention. Let these lunch ideas be a source of inspiration as you embark on your journey towards a healthier and more vibrant lifestyle, one delicious meal at a time.

3.1. Balanced Salad Options

Salads are a lunchtime staple celebrated for their versatility, freshness, and nutritional prowess. When crafted with care and attention, salads have the power to satisfy hunger, tantalize the taste buds, and nourish the body with a wealth of vitamins, minerals, and fiber. In this exploration of balanced salad options, we uncover a spectrum of creative combinations, vibrant flavors, and satisfying textures that elevate salads from simple side dishes to hearty main courses worthy of center stage.

Building a Nutrient-Dense Foundation

At the heart of every balanced salad lies a foundation of nutrient-dense ingredients that form the base of the dish and provide a wealth of essential vitamins, minerals, and antioxidants. Start with a bed of leafy greens such as spinach, kale, arugula, or mixed lettuces to provide a crisp and refreshing backdrop for your salad.

Incorporate a variety of colorful vegetables such as tomatoes, cucumbers, bell peppers, carrots, and radishes to add crunch, flavor, and visual appeal to your salad. These nutrient-rich vegetables not only contribute to a satisfying texture but also provide a host of health benefits, from supporting digestion to boosting immune function.

Protein Powerhouses

To transform your salad into a satisfying and satiating meal, incorporate protein-rich ingredients that provide long-lasting energy and promote muscle repair and growth. Opt for lean sources of protein such as grilled chicken breast, turkey, tofu, tempeh, or legumes to add substance and depth to your salad.

Experiment with different protein sources to keep your salads exciting and varied, from marinated grilled shrimp and seared tuna to hard-boiled eggs and quinoa. By combining protein with fiber-rich vegetables and healthy fats, you can create a balanced and nutritious meal that satisfies hunger and supports optimal health.

Healthy Fats and Flavor Enhancers

To enhance the flavor and nutritional profile of your balanced salad, incorporate healthy fats and flavor enhancers that add richness, depth, and complexity to the dish. Add slices of creamy avocado, toasted nuts, seeds, or crumbled cheese such as feta, goat cheese, or blue cheese to provide a satisfying texture and savory flavor to your salad.

Drizzle your salad with a homemade vinaigrette or dressing made from heart-healthy oils such as olive oil, avocado oil, or flaxseed oil, combined with tangy vinegars, citrus juices, herbs, and spices. Experiment with different flavor combinations to create a dressing that complements the ingredients in your salad while enhancing their natural flavors.

Whole Grains and Fiber-Rich Additions

For added texture, fiber, and satiety, consider incorporating whole grains and fiber-rich additions into your balanced salad. Add cooked grains such as quinoa, farro, brown rice, or barley to provide a hearty and satisfying element that complements the other ingredients in your salad.Incorporate fiber-rich additions such as beans, lentils, chickpeas, or edamame to add bulk, protein, and fiber to your salad while keeping carbohydrate levels in check. These plant-based additions not only contribute to a feeling of fullness and satisfaction but also provide a steady source of energy and support digestive health.

Customization and Creative Combinations

The beauty of balanced salad options lies in their versatility and adaptability to suit individual tastes, preferences, and dietary needs. Experiment with different combinations of ingredients, flavors, and textures to create salads that reflect your culinary creativity and personal preferences.

From Mediterranean-inspired salads with olives, sun-dried tomatoes, and artichokes to Asian-inspired salads with sesame ginger dressing, tofu, and crunchy cabbage, the possibilities for creative combinations are endless. Customize your salad to suit your nutritional goals and flavor preferences, whether you prefer a light and refreshing option or a hearty and satisfying meal.

Conclusion

In conclusion, balanced salad options offer a delicious and nutritious way to enjoy a satisfying and satisfying meal that supports your health and well-being. By incorporating nutrient-dense ingredients, protein powerhouses, healthy fats, fiber-rich additions, and creative flavor combinations, you can create salads that delight the senses and nourish the body.

With a multitude of ingredients, textures, and flavors at your disposal, balanced salad options invite you to explore the vibrant world of culinary creativity and customization. Whether you're looking for a light and refreshing option or a hearty and satisfying meal, there's a balanced salad option to suit every taste and lifestyle, making it easy and enjoyable to incorporate nutritious, diabetes-friendly meals into your lunchtime routine.

3.2. Flavorful Soup Recipes

Soup, with its comforting warmth and rich flavors, stands as a timeless lunchtime favorite, cherished for its versatility and nourishing qualities. From hearty stews to light broths, flavorful soups offer a satisfying meal that warms the body and soothes the soul. In this exploration of flavorful soup recipes, we delve into a variety of ingredients, seasonings, and cooking techniques to create soups that tantalize the taste buds and satisfy hunger cravings.

Nourishing Bone Broth Base

At the heart of many flavorful soup recipes lies a nourishing bone broth base, rich in vitamins, minerals, and amino acids that support overall health and well-being. Start by simmering bones—such as chicken, beef, or turkey—with aromatic vegetables, herbs, and spices in water to create a flavorful and nutrient-rich broth. Allow the broth to simmer low and slow for several hours to extract the maximum amount of flavor and nutrients from the bones and vegetables. Strain the broth to remove any solids, then use it as the foundation for a variety of flavorful soup recipes, from classic chicken noodle soup to hearty beef stew.

Seasonal Vegetable Soups

One of the joys of soup-making lies in its adaptability to seasonal ingredients, allowing you to create flavorful soups using fresh, seasonal produce at its peak of ripeness and flavor. During the cooler months, opt for root vegetables such as carrots, potatoes, and squash to create hearty and comforting soups that warm the body and soul.

In the spring and summer months, take advantage of vibrant seasonal vegetables such as tomatoes, zucchini, bell peppers, and green beans to create light and refreshing soups that celebrate the bounty of the season. Experiment with different combinations of vegetables, herbs, and spices to create soups that reflect the flavors of the season and satisfy your taste buds.

Global-Inspired Flavors

Expand your culinary horizons by exploring global-inspired flavors and ingredients in your soup recipes, drawing inspiration from cuisines around the world to create bold and flavorful dishes. From spicy Thai curry soups to aromatic Moroccan tagines, the possibilities for global-inspired soups are endless. Experiment with different spices, herbs, and condiments to create complex and nuanced flavor profiles that transport you to far-off lands with each spoonful. Whether you're craving the rich umami flavors of Japanese miso soup or the fiery heat of Mexican tortilla soup, there's a global-inspired soup recipe to suit every palate and preference.

Creamy and Comforting Creations

Indulge in creamy and comforting soup creations that satisfy both the palate and the soul, offering a luxurious and indulgent dining experience that's perfect for chilly days and cozy evenings. Incorporate ingredients such as cream, coconut milk, or puréed vegetables to create rich and velvety textures that envelop the taste buds in decadent goodness. Add depth and complexity to your creamy soups with the addition of aromatic spices, herbs, and flavorings such as garlic, ginger, curry powder, or fresh herbs. Whether you're craving the classic comfort of creamy tomato soup or the exotic allure of coconut curry soup, creamy and comforting soup creations offer a satisfying and indulgent meal that's sure to warm your heart.

Nutrient-Dense Additions

Boost the nutritional value of your flavorful soup recipes by incorporating nutrient-dense additions such as legumes, whole grains, and lean proteins that add texture, flavor, and satiety to your soup. Add cooked beans, lentils, or chickpeas to create hearty and filling soups that are packed with fiber and protein.

Incorporate whole grains such as quinoa, barley, or brown rice to add a satisfying chewiness and nutty flavor to your soup while providing essential vitamins, minerals, and antioxidants. Add lean proteins such as diced chicken breast, turkey, or tofu to create soups that satisfy hunger cravings and support muscle repair and growth.

Conclusion

In conclusion, flavorful soup recipes offer a delicious and nourishing option for lunch that satisfies both the palate and the body. By exploring a variety of ingredients, seasonings, and cooking techniques, you can create soups that delight the senses and nourish the soul.

Whether you're craving the comforting warmth of a seasonal vegetable soup, the bold flavors of a global-inspired creation, or the creamy indulgence of a luxurious bisque, there's a flavorful soup recipe to suit every taste and preference. With nutrient-dense additions, seasonal vegetables, and global-inspired flavors, flavorful soup recipes invite you to embrace the joy of soup-making and enjoy a satisfying and nourishing meal that's perfect for any occasion.

3.3. Wraps and Sandwiches for Diabetics

Wraps and sandwiches offer a convenient and portable lunchtime option that's perfect for those with busy schedules or on-the-go lifestyles. When crafted with diabetes management in mind, wraps and sandwiches can be transformed into delicious and satisfying meals that provide balanced nutrition without causing spikes in blood sugar levels. In this exploration of wraps and sandwiches for diabetics, we uncover a variety of creative combinations, wholesome ingredients, and flavor-packed fillings that make lunchtime both enjoyable and nutritious.

Choosing the Right Bread or Wrap

The foundation of any wrap or sandwich lies in selecting the right type of bread or wrap that's suitable for a diabetic-friendly meal. Opt for whole grain or whole wheat breads that are high in fiber and low in added sugars to help stabilize blood sugar levels and promote satiety.

Alternatively, choose whole grain or whole wheat wraps, tortillas, or flatbreads that offer a lighter and more portable option for those who prefer a wrap-style sandwich. Look for options that are labeled as low-carb or high-fiber to ensure that your wrap or sandwich fits within your dietary guidelines for managing diabetes.

Incorporating Lean Proteins

To create a satisfying and balanced wrap or sandwich, incorporate lean sources of protein that provide essential amino acids while keeping saturated fat and cholesterol levels in check. Choose lean proteins such as grilled chicken breast, turkey, roast beef, or tofu to add substance and flavor to your wrap or sandwich.

Consider incorporating plant-based proteins such as beans, lentils, chickpeas, or hummus for a vegetarian-friendly option that's rich in fiber and nutrients. These protein-packed fillings not only provide a satisfying texture and flavor but also help to promote fullness and stabilize blood sugar levels throughout the day.

Adding Crunchy Vegetables and Fresh Greens

Enhance the nutritional value and texture of your wrap or sandwich by incorporating crunchy vegetables and fresh greens that provide a burst of color, flavor, and essential vitamins and minerals. Add slices of crisp lettuce, spinach, or kale to provide a refreshing and nutrient-rich base for your wrap or sandwich.

Incorporate a variety of colorful vegetables such as tomatoes, cucumbers, bell peppers, onions, and carrots to add crunch, sweetness, and visual appeal to your wrap or sandwich. These fiber-rich additions not only contribute to a satisfying texture but also help to promote digestive health and overall well-being.

Incorporating Healthy Fats and Flavor Enhancers

Boost the flavor and nutritional value of your wrap or sandwich by incorporating healthy fats and flavor enhancers that add richness, depth, and complexity to the dish. Add slices of creamy avocado, spreads of nut butter, or drizzles of olive oil to provide a satisfying texture and savory flavor to your wrap or sandwich.

Incorporate flavorful condiments such as mustard, salsa, pesto, or tzatziki to add zing and zest to your wrap or sandwich without adding excess calories or carbohydrates. Experiment with different herbs, spices, and seasonings to create custom flavor profiles that suit your taste preferences and dietary needs.

Customization and Creative Combinations

The beauty of wraps and sandwiches lies in their versatility and adaptability to suit individual tastes, preferences, and dietary needs. Experiment with different combinations of ingredients, fillings, and condiments to create wraps and sandwiches that reflect your culinary creativity and personal preferences.

From classic combinations such as turkey and cranberry sauce to more exotic options like Thai chicken lettuce wraps or Mediterranean veggie wraps, the possibilities for creative combinations are endless. Customize your wrap or sandwich to suit your nutritional goals and flavor preferences, whether you prefer a light and refreshing option or a hearty and satisfying meal.

Conclusion

In conclusion, wraps, and sandwiches for diabetics offer a delicious and convenient lunchtime option that's both satisfying and nutritious. By choosing the right bread or wrap, incorporating lean proteins, adding crunchy vegetables and fresh greens, incorporating healthy fats and flavor enhancers, and experimenting with creative combinations, you can create wraps and sandwiches that cater to your dietary needs while tantalizing your taste buds.

Whether you're craving a classic turkey and cheese sandwich, a veggie-packed wrap with hummus, or a protein-rich lettuce wrap with grilled chicken, wraps, and sandwiches for diabetics offer a versatile and delicious way to enjoy a satisfying lunch that supports your health and well-being. With a little creativity and ingenuity, you can transform ordinary wraps and sandwiches into flavorful and nutritious meals that make lunchtime something to look forward to.

Conclusion

In conclusion, lunchtime offers an opportunity to nourish the body and delight the senses with delicious and diabetes-friendly meals that prioritize balance, flavor, and satisfaction. By incorporating wholesome ingredients, creative flavor combinations, and mindful cooking techniques, these lunch ideas provide a roadmap for enjoying meals that support blood sugar management and promote overall well-being. As we conclude our exploration of lunch ideas, we're reminded of the power of food to nourish, energize, and uplift both body and spirit. Whether you're enjoying a hearty salad packed with seasonal vegetables, savoring a comforting bowl of soup on a chilly day, or indulging in a satisfying wrap or sandwich, may each bite be a celebration of health, vitality, and joy. With a wealth of options to choose from, lunchtime becomes an opportunity to nourish yourself with meals that not only fuel your body, but also nourish your soul. Let these lunch ideas inspire you to embrace the pleasure of cooking and eating with intention, making every meal a delicious and fulfilling experience that supports your journey towards better health and well-being.

Chapter 4

"Dinner Dishes"

Introduction

Welcome to the vibrant world of dinner dishes, where flavor, nutrition, and convenience come together to create delicious meals that satisfy the body and soul. In this chapter, we explore a variety of dinner dishes designed to elevate your dining experience, from lean protein entrées and vegetable-packed stir-fries to wholesome one-pot meals that bring comfort and nourishment to the table. Dinner is a time to unwind, connect with loved ones, and nourish ourselves with wholesome food that fuels our bodies and delights our senses. Whether you're a busy professional juggling multiple responsibilities or a home cook seeking inspiration in the kitchen, this chapter offers a wealth of culinary creations to suit your taste preferences, dietary needs, and lifestyle. Prepare to embark on a culinary journey filled with bold flavors, fresh ingredients, and creative cooking techniques that will transform your dinner routine into a culinary adventure. From quick and easy weeknight meals to leisurely weekend feasts, these dinner dishes are sure to become cherished favorites in your repertoire, providing sustenance and satisfaction with every bite.

4.1. Lean Protein Entrées

In the realm of dinner dishes, lean protein entrées stand as pillars of nutrition, offering a hearty and satisfying meal that supports muscle health, satiety, and overall well-being. In this exploration of lean protein entrées, we delve into a variety of delicious and nutritious options that cater to a range of tastes and dietary preferences, providing ample protein without excess fat or carbohydrates. From succulent poultry and tender seafood to wholesome plant-based options, these lean protein entrées are sure to elevate your dinner table with flavor and nourishment.

Poultry Perfection

Poultry, such as chicken and turkey, reigns supreme in the realm of lean protein entrées, offering a versatile canvas for culinary creativity and flavor exploration. Opt for skinless, boneless cuts of chicken breast or turkey breast to minimize saturated fat and calories while maximizing protein content. Experiment with different cooking techniques, from grilling and baking to sautéing and roasting, to create tender and succulent poultry entrées that are bursting with flavor. Marinate chicken breasts in a tangy citrus marinade, or rub turkey cutlets with a savory spice blend for a delicious and aromatic meal that's sure to impress.

Sustainable Seafood Selections

Seafood provides an excellent source of lean protein, along with essential omega-3 fatty acids that support heart health and brain function. Choose fatty fish such as salmon, mackerel, or trout for a rich and flavorful entrée that's packed with protein and healthy fats. For a lighter option, opt for leaner varieties such as cod, tilapia, or shrimp, which offer a mild flavor and delicate texture that pairs well with a variety of seasonings and sauces. Whether grilled, baked, or broiled, seafood entrées offer a delicious and nutritious addition to any dinner menu.

Plant-Powered Options

For those following a plant-based diet or looking to incorporate more meatless meals into their routine, plant-powered options provide a satisfying and nutritious alternative to traditional protein sources. Lentils, beans, tofu, and tempeh offer ample protein along with fiber, vitamins, and minerals that support overall health and well-being. Experiment with different plant-based proteins to create hearty and satisfying entrées such as lentil shepherd's pie, black bean tacos, or tofu stir-fry. Incorporate a variety of vegetables, herbs, and spices to add flavor and texture to your plant-powered creations, making them both delicious and nutritious.

Innovative Ingredient Combinations

Elevate your lean protein entrées with innovative ingredient combinations that tantalize the taste buds and add depth and complexity to your meals. Pair grilled chicken breast with a tangy mango salsa for a burst of tropical flavor, or top baked salmon with a creamy dill yogurt sauce for a refreshing and aromatic twist. Experiment with global-inspired flavors and cuisines, from Mediterranean-style chicken skewers with tzatziki sauce to Asian-inspired sesame-crusted tuna steaks. Incorporate a variety of herbs, spices, and condiments to create custom flavor profiles that reflect your culinary preferences and dietary needs.

Conclusion

In conclusion, lean protein entrées offer a delicious and nutritious way to elevate your dinner table with flavor, satisfaction, and nourishment. Whether you prefer poultry, seafood, or plant-based options, there's a lean protein entrée to suit every taste and dietary preference.

By incorporating wholesome ingredients, innovative cooking techniques, and creative flavor combinations, you can create lean protein entrées that satisfy both the palate and the body. With a focus on balance, variety, and culinary creativity, lean protein entrées are sure to become a staple of your dinner rotation, providing delicious and nutritious meals that support your health and well-being.

4.2. Vegetable-Packed Stir-Fries

Stir-fries are a beloved staple in many households, celebrated for their vibrant flavors, quick cooking time, and versatility in incorporating a variety of vegetables. In this exploration of vegetable-packed stir-fries, we dive into the art of stir-frying, exploring techniques, ingredient combinations, and flavor profiles that elevate this humble dish into a nutritious and satisfying dinner option.

The Art of Stir-Frying

At the heart of every great stir-fry lies the art of stir-frying itself—a cooking technique that involves quickly cooking bite-sized pieces of ingredients in a hot pan or wok with a small amount of oil over high heat. Stir-frying allows for the preservation of nutrients and vibrant colors in vegetables while creating a deliciously charred and caramelized exterior. To achieve the perfect stir-fry, it's essential to have all your ingredients prepped and ready to go before you start cooking. This includes washing, chopping, and measuring out your vegetables, proteins, aromatics, and sauces, ensuring that everything is within arm's reach once you start cooking.

Building Flavor with Aromatics and Sauces

Aromatics such as garlic, ginger, onions, and shallots play a crucial role in infusing stir-fries with depth and complexity of flavor. Begin by sautéing these aromatics in a small amount of oil until fragrant, releasing their essential oils and building a flavorful base for the stir-fry.

Sauces are another essential component of a delicious stir-fry, providing seasoning, umami richness, and a glossy coating to the ingredients. Common stir-fry sauces include soy sauce, oyster sauce, hoisin sauce, and chili sauce, which can be customized to suit your taste preferences and dietary needs. Experiment with different combinations of sauces, balancing salty, sweet, sour, and spicy flavors to create a harmonious and well-rounded stir-fry sauce.

Incorporating a Variety of Vegetables

One of the hallmarks of a vegetable-packed stir-fry is, of course, the vegetables themselves. Stir-fries offer a fantastic opportunity to incorporate a colorful array of vegetables, from crunchy bell peppers and snap peas to tender broccoli florets and earthy mushrooms.

When selecting vegetables for your stir-fry, aim for a diverse mix of colors, textures, and flavors to create a visually appealing and nutritionally balanced dish. Consider incorporating seasonal vegetables for optimal freshness and flavor, adapting your stir-fry recipe to reflect the bounty of the season.

Balancing Texture and Cooking Times

Achieving the perfect texture in a stir-fry requires careful attention to cooking times and techniques. Begin by stir-frying harder vegetables such as carrots and broccoli first, allowing them to soften slightly before adding quicker-cooking vegetables such as bell peppers and snow peas. To maintain crispness and freshness, avoid overcooking the vegetables, opting instead for a quick and high-heat cooking method that preserves their natural crunch and vibrancy. Stir-fry in small batches if necessary, ensuring that each ingredient cooks evenly and retains its individual texture and flavor.

Customizing with Protein Options

While stir-fries are traditionally vegetable-centric, adding protein can elevate them into a complete and satisfying meal. Lean proteins such as chicken breast, shrimp, tofu, or tempeh can be incorporated into stir-fries, adding a hearty and satiating element to the dish. When adding protein to your stir-fry, cook it separately before combining it with the vegetables and sauce, ensuring that it cooks evenly and develops a golden crust or tender texture. Alternatively, marinate the protein in a flavorful sauce before stir-frying, allowing it to absorb the flavors and infuse the dish with richness and depth.

Garnishing and Serving Suggestions

Garnishes are the finishing touch that adds visual appeal, texture, and flavor to a vegetable-packed stir-fry. Sprinkle toasted sesame seeds, chopped peanuts, or fresh herbs such as cilantro or green onions over the finished dish for added crunch and freshness. Serve your stir-fry piping hot alongside steamed rice, quinoa, or noodles for a complete and satisfying meal. Alternatively, wrap the stir-fry in lettuce leaves or cabbage leaves for a low-carb option, or spoon it over a bed of mixed greens for a lighter and refreshing twist.

Conclusion

In conclusion, vegetable-packed stir-fries offer a delicious and nutritious dinner option that's both quick and easy to prepare. By mastering the art of stir-frying, building flavor with aromatics and sauces, incorporating a variety of vegetables, balancing texture and cooking times, customizing with protein options, and garnishing with flair, you can create stir-fries that delight the senses and nourish the body. Whether you're a novice cook or a seasoned chef, vegetable-packed stir-fries invite you to explore the vibrant world of Asian-inspired cuisine, embracing bold flavors, fresh ingredients, and creative cooking techniques. With endless possibilities for customization and adaptation, stir-fries are sure to become a favorite go-to dinner dish in your culinary repertoire, providing delicious and satisfying meals for you and your loved ones to enjoy.

4.3. Wholesome One-Pot Meals

One-pot meals are a lifesaver for busy individuals seeking nourishing and convenient dinner options without sacrificing flavor or nutrition. In this exploration of wholesome one-pot meals, we delve into the world of hearty and satisfying dishes that can be prepared with minimal effort and cleanup, making them perfect for busy weeknights or lazy weekends alike.

The Beauty of One-Pot Cooking

At the heart of every wholesome one-pot meal lies the beauty of one-pot cooking—an approach that involves combining all ingredients into a single pot or pan and allowing them to cook together, melding flavors and textures into a harmonious and satisfying dish.

One-pot meals offer the convenience of minimal prep and cleanup, making them ideal for busy households or those seeking to streamline their cooking routine.

Versatility and Adaptability

One of the greatest strengths of one-pot meals is their versatility and adaptability to a wide range of ingredients and dietary preferences. Whether you prefer hearty stews, comforting casseroles, or aromatic curries, there's a one-pot meal to suit every taste and craving. Experiment with different combinations of proteins, grains, vegetables, and aromatics to create custom one-pot meals that reflect your culinary preferences and dietary needs. Incorporate seasonal ingredients for optimal freshness and flavor, adapting your recipes to showcase the bounty of the season.

Balanced Nutrition

Despite their simplicity, one-pot meals can be incredibly nutritious, providing a balanced mix of protein, carbohydrates, and vegetables in every bite. Lean proteins such as chicken, turkey, or tofu can serve as the foundation of your one-pot meal, while whole grains such as quinoa, brown rice, or farro add fiber and complex carbohydrates to keep you feeling satisfied. Load up on colorful vegetables such as bell peppers, spinach, carrots, and broccoli to boost the nutritional content of your one-pot meal, providing essential vitamins, minerals, and antioxidants that support overall health and well-being. Don't forget to incorporate healthy fats such as olive oil, avocado, or nuts to add richness and flavor to your dishes.

Flavorful Seasonings and Broths

The key to a delicious one-pot meal lies in the seasonings and broths used to flavor the dish. Experiment with a variety of herbs, spices, and condiments to create custom flavor profiles that tantalize the taste buds and elevate your meal to new heights. From aromatic garlic and ginger to warming cumin and paprika, the possibilities for seasoning your one-pot meals are endless. Consider using homemade or low-sodium broths to control the salt content of your dish, or opt for flavorful alternatives such as coconut milk or tomato sauce for added depth and richness.

Effortless Preparation and Cleanup

One of the greatest advantages of one-pot meals is their effortless preparation and cleanup. With minimal chopping, sautéing, and stirring required, one-pot meals can be assembled in a matter of minutes, allowing you to spend less time in the kitchen and more time enjoying your meal with loved ones. After enjoying your delicious one-pot meal, cleanup is a breeze with only one pot or pan to wash, saving you time and effort on dishwashing duty. Simply soak the pot in warm, soapy water while you dine, then give it a quick scrub and rinse once you're finished—no need for a sink full of dirty dishes.

Family-Friendly Favorites

One-pot meals are perfect for feeding the whole family, offering a convenient and satisfying option that's sure to please even the pickiest eaters. Whether you're serving up a hearty chili, a creamy pasta dish, or a fragrant curry, one-pot meals bring everyone together around the dinner table for a cozy and comforting mealtime experience.

Get the kids involved in meal prep by letting them help chop vegetables, measure ingredients, or stir the pot—making dinner a fun and interactive activity for the whole family. Encourage creativity by allowing family members to customize their one-pot meals with their favorite toppings or garnishes, ensuring that everyone finds something to love.

Conclusion

In conclusion, wholesome one-pot meals offer a delicious and convenient dinner option that's perfect for busy individuals and families alike. With their versatility, adaptability, and balanced nutrition, one-pot meals provide a satisfying and nourishing mealtime solution that requires minimal effort and cleanup. Whether you're craving a comforting stew, a hearty casserole, or a flavorful curry, there's a one-pot meal to suit every taste and occasion. Embrace the simplicity and convenience of one-pot cooking, and let these wholesome meals become a staple of your dinner rotation, providing delicious and satisfying meals for you and your loved ones to enjoy.

Conclusion

In conclusion, dinner dishes play a vital role in our lives, nourishing our bodies and bringing joy to our dining experiences. From the simplicity of lean protein entrées to the versatility of vegetable-packed stir-fries and the comforting embrace of wholesome one-pot meals, the possibilities for dinner are endless. As we navigate the demands of modern life, it's essential to prioritize wholesome and nutritious meals that support our health and well-being. By embracing the diverse array of dinner dishes presented in this chapter, we can cultivate a deeper connection to the food we eat and the nourishment it provides, fostering a greater appreciation for the culinary arts and the role they play in our lives. So let us raise our forks and toast to the magic of dinner dishes—to the flavors that tantalize our taste buds, the ingredients that nourish our bodies, and the memories created around the dinner table. May these dishes inspire creativity, foster connection, and bring joy to our lives for years to come.

Introduction

Welcome to Chapter 5: Snack Time Solutions. In this chapter, we'll explore a variety of nutritious and delicious snack options to keep you fueled and satisfied throughout the day. Whether you're looking for a quick bite between meals, a pre-workout boost, or a healthy option to satisfy your sweet tooth, we've got you covered with a range of snack ideas that are easy to make, portable, and bursting with flavor. Snacking plays a crucial role in maintaining energy levels, managing hunger, and supporting overall health and well-being. However, not all snacks are created equal, and it's essential to choose options that provide a balance of nutrients to keep you feeling your best. That's why we've curated a collection of snack recipes that are not only tasty and satisfying but also nutritious and wholesome. From homemade energy bars packed with protein and fiber to veggie sticks with creamy dips bursting with vitamins and minerals, these snack time solutions are designed to fuel your body with the nutrients it needs to thrive. Say goodbye to processed snacks loaded with added sugars, artificial flavors, and preservatives, and say hello to delicious, nourishing snacks that you can feel good about enjoying.

Chapter 5

"Snack Time Solutions"

5.1. Nutritious Trail Mixes

Trail mixes are a beloved snack choice for outdoor enthusiasts, busy professionals, and anyone in need of a quick and satisfying energy boost. Combining a variety of nuts, seeds, dried fruits, and other tasty morsels, trail mixes offer a convenient and portable source of nutrition that's perfect for on-the-go snacking. In this section, we'll explore the art of creating nutritious trail mixes that tantalize the taste buds while providing a balanced mix of nutrients to fuel your adventures.

The Foundation: Nuts and Seeds

At the heart of every nutritious trail mix lies the foundation of nuts and seeds, providing essential fats, protein, and fiber to keep you feeling full and satisfied. Opt for a variety of nuts and seeds to create a diverse mix of flavors and textures, including almonds, walnuts, cashews, peanuts, pumpkin seeds, sunflower seeds, and sesame seeds. Nuts and seeds are nutritional powerhouses, packed with heart-healthy fats, vitamins, minerals, and antioxidants that support overall health and well-being. They're also a great source of energy, making them an ideal snack choice for sustained fuel during long hikes, bike rides, or busy days at work.

Adding Sweetness: Dried Fruits

To balance out the savory and salty flavors of nuts and seeds, dried fruits are added to trail mixes to provide natural sweetness and chewy texture. Choose from a variety of dried fruits such as raisins, cranberries, apricots, cherries, mangoes, and pineapple, ensuring a colorful and flavorful mix that appeals to your taste preferences. Dried fruits are not only delicious but also rich in vitamins, minerals, and dietary fiber, making them a nutritious addition to any trail mix. However, it's important to enjoy them in moderation due to their concentrated sugar content. Aim for a balance of nuts, seeds, and dried fruits to keep your trail mix both tasty and nutritious.

Boosting Flavor and Nutrition: Additional Ingredients

In addition to nuts, seeds, and dried fruits, trail mixes can be enhanced with a variety of additional ingredients to boost flavor, nutrition, and texture. Consider adding ingredients such as dark chocolate chips, coconut flakes, whole-grain cereal, pretzel sticks, or popcorn for added crunch and variety. Dark chocolate adds a decadent touch to trail mixes, while providing antioxidants and flavonoids that support heart health and cognitive function. Coconut flakes offer a tropical flair and a dose of healthy fats, while whole-grain cereal and popcorn contribute fiber and crunch without excess calories or added sugars.

Customizing to Suit Your Taste

The beauty of trail mixes lies in their versatility and adaptability to suit your taste preferences and dietary needs. Feel free to experiment with different combinations of nuts, seeds, dried fruits, and additional ingredients to create custom trail mixes that reflect your personal flavor profile and nutritional goals.

Whether you prefer a sweet and savory mix, a spicy and tangy blend, or a simple and classic combination, the possibilities for trail mixes are endless. Get creative in the kitchen, and don't be afraid to try new flavor combinations and ingredient pairings to discover your perfect trail mix recipe.

Portion Control and Storage Tips

While trail mixes are undeniably delicious and nutritious, it's essential to practice portion control to avoid overindulgence. Stick to a serving size of around ¼ to ½ cup of trail mix per serving, depending on your calorie needs and activity level. To keep your trail mixes fresh and flavorful, store them in an airtight container in a cool, dry place away from direct sunlight. Avoid storing trail mixes in the refrigerator or freezer, as the moisture can cause the nuts and seeds to become stale or soggy.

Conclusion

In conclusion, nutritious trail mixes offer a convenient and satisfying snack option that's perfect for fueling your adventures and satisfying your cravings. By combining a variety of nuts, seeds, dried fruits, and additional ingredients, you can create custom trail mixes that provide a balanced mix of nutrients, flavors, and textures to keep you energized and satisfied throughout the day. Whether you're hitting the trails, powering through a busy workday, or simply seeking a tasty and nutritious snack, trail mixes are sure to become a staple in your snack rotation. With endless possibilities for customization and creativity, trail mixes invite you to explore new flavors, experiment with different ingredients, and discover your perfect blend of trail mix bliss.

5.2. Veggie Sticks with Dips

When it comes to healthy snacking, few options rival the simplicity and satisfaction of veggie sticks paired with delicious dips. Bursting with flavor, color, and nutrition, this snack offers a delightful combination of crunchy vegetables and creamy dips that is sure to tantalize your taste buds and nourish your body. In this section, we'll explore the art of creating veggie sticks with dips that are both delicious and nutritious, providing a satisfying snack solution for any occasion.

Crunchy and Colorful Veggie Sticks

The foundation of any veggie sticks and dip platter lies in the selection of fresh, crunchy vegetables that serve as the perfect vehicles for scooping up creamy dips. Opt for a colorful array of vegetables to create visual appeal and maximize nutritional variety. Some popular choices include:

- Crisp carrot sticks

- Crunchy celery stalks

- Vibrant bell pepper strips (red, yellow, or green)

- Juicy cucumber slices

- Tender snap peas

- Crisp broccoli or cauliflower florets

By incorporating a variety of vegetables, you not only enhance the visual appeal of your snack but also ensure a diverse range of vitamins, minerals, and antioxidants to support overall health and well-being.

Creamy and Flavorful Dips

Complement your crunchy veggie sticks with an assortment of creamy and flavorful dips that add depth and richness to every bite. Whether you prefer classic favorites or adventurous flavor combinations, there's a dip to suit every taste preference and dietary need. Some popular dip options include:

- Classic hummus, made from chickpeas, tahini, lemon juice, and garlic

- Creamy avocado dip, featuring ripe avocado, lime juice, cilantro, and spices

- Tangy tzatziki, a Greek yogurt-based dip flavored with cucumber, garlic, and dill

- Spicy salsa, made from ripe tomatoes, onions, jalapeños, and cilantro

- Nutty almond butter or cashew butter, perfect for dipping crisp apple slices

Experiment with different dip recipes and flavor profiles to discover your favorites, and don't be afraid to get creative by adding fresh herbs, spices, or citrus zest to customize your dips to suit your taste preferences.

Nutritious and Satisfying Snacking

Veggie sticks with dips offer a nutritious and satisfying snacking solution that's perfect for any time of day. Packed with fiber, vitamins, minerals, and antioxidants, vegetables provide essential nutrients that support overall health and well-being. Meanwhile, creamy dips add satiating fats and proteins that help keep hunger at bay and provide sustained energy throughout the day. By choosing whole, minimally processed ingredients for your veggie sticks and dips, you can feel good about indulging in this delicious snack without worrying about excess calories, additives, or preservatives. Plus, the combination of crunchy vegetables and creamy dips offers a satisfying sensory experience that satisfies cravings and promotes mindful eating.

Convenient and Portable Snack Option

In addition to being nutritious and satisfying, veggie sticks with dips are also incredibly convenient and portable, making them an ideal snack option for busy individuals on the go. Whether you're packing a lunch for work, heading out for a picnic, or simply craving a healthy snack at home, veggie sticks with dips are easy to prepare and transport, allowing you to enjoy fresh, wholesome snacking wherever you go. To make your veggie sticks and dips even more convenient, consider prepping and portioning them ahead of time for grab-and-go snacking. Pack individual servings of veggies and dips in reusable containers or snack bags, making it easy to enjoy a nutritious snack whenever hunger strikes.

Family-Friendly Snacking

Veggie sticks with dips aren't just for adults—they're also a hit with kids of all ages. Get the whole family involved in snack time by inviting them to help wash, chop, and assemble the veggies, encouraging them to try new flavors and textures along the way. With a variety of colorful vegetables and flavorful dips to choose from, veggie sticks with dips make healthy snacking fun and exciting for everyone. Encourage kids to get creative with their veggie stick combinations, allowing them to mix and match different vegetables and dips to create their own custom snack creations. By involving children in the snack preparation process, you not only promote healthy eating habits but also foster a sense of independence and culinary exploration that will serve them well throughout their lives.

Conclusion

In conclusion, veggie sticks with dips offer a delicious, nutritious, and satisfying snacking solution that's perfect for any occasion. With their crunchy textures, vibrant colors, and creamy flavors, veggie sticks and dips provide a sensory experience that delights the palate and nourishes the body. Whether you're enjoying them as a midday pick-me-up, a pre-dinner appetizer, or a post-workout refuel, veggie sticks with dips are sure to satisfy your cravings and fuel your body with essential nutrients. So next time you're in need of a healthy and delicious snack, reach for a platter of veggie sticks with dips and savor the goodness of fresh, wholesome ingredients.

5.3. Homemade Energy Bars

In today's fast-paced world, having convenient and nutritious snack options on hand is essential for maintaining energy levels and supporting overall well-being. Homemade energy bars are a popular choice among health-conscious individuals seeking a quick and satisfying snack that's packed with wholesome ingredients and free from artificial additives. In this section, we'll delve into the world of homemade energy bars, exploring how to create delicious and nutritious bars that provide sustained energy and satisfaction throughout the day.

The Appeal of Homemade Energy Bars

Homemade energy bars have gained popularity in recent years as people seek healthier alternatives to store-bought granola bars and protein bars, which often contain high levels of added sugars, preservatives, and artificial ingredients. By making energy bars at home, you have full control over the ingredients, allowing you to customize the recipe to suit your taste preferences and dietary needs. Not only are homemade energy bars delicious and nutritious, but they're also incredibly versatile, allowing you to experiment with different flavor combinations and ingredient variations to create your perfect snack. Whether you prefer chewy fruit and nut bars, crunchy granola bars, or protein-packed power bars, the options are endless when it comes to homemade energy bars.

Key Ingredients for Homemade Energy Bars

The beauty of homemade energy bars lies in their simplicity and flexibility. While the exact ingredients may vary depending on the recipe, most homemade energy bars are made with a base of nutritious ingredients that provide a balance of carbohydrates, protein, and healthy fats to fuel your body and satisfy your hunger. Some key ingredients commonly found in homemade energy bars include:

- Rolled oats or quinoa flakes: These whole grains provide complex carbohydrates for sustained energy and fiber to support digestive health.

- Nuts and seeds: Almonds, walnuts, cashews, pumpkin seeds, and chia seeds are popular choices for adding protein, healthy fats, and crunch to energy bars.

- Dried fruits: Dates, figs, apricots, and raisins add natural sweetness and chewy texture to energy bars while providing vitamins, minerals, and antioxidants.

- Nut butter or seed butter: Peanut butter, almond butter, and tahini are often used as binding agents and flavor enhancers in energy bar recipes, adding richness and creaminess to the bars.

- Sweeteners: Natural sweeteners such as honey, maple syrup, or agave nectar may be used sparingly to enhance the flavor of energy bars without relying on refined sugars.

Customizing Your Energy Bars

One of the greatest advantages of making energy bars at home is the ability to customize the recipe to suit your taste preferences and dietary restrictions. Whether you're vegan, gluten-free, or following a specific eating plan, you can adapt energy bar recipes to meet your needs by swapping out ingredients and adjusting the quantities accordingly.

For example, if you're vegan, you can use plant-based protein powders or nut butter in place of whey protein and honey. If you're gluten-free, you can use gluten-free oats or quinoa flakes instead of traditional rolled oats. And if you're watching your sugar intake, you can reduce or omit the sweeteners altogether and rely on the natural sweetness of dried fruits or a touch of cinnamon or vanilla extract to enhance the flavor of your bars.

Preparing and Storing Homemade Energy Bars

Making homemade energy bars is relatively simple and requires minimal equipment. Most recipes involve combining the ingredients in a food processor or mixing bowl, pressing the mixture into a baking dish or mold, and then chilling or baking until set. Once cooled, the bars can be cut into individual servings and stored in an airtight container in the refrigerator or freezer for long-term storage.

When it comes to storing homemade energy bars, it's essential to keep them in a cool, dry place away from direct sunlight to prevent them from becoming too soft or sticky. If you prefer a firmer texture, you can store the bars in the refrigerator, where they will stay fresh for up to two weeks. Alternatively, you can store them in the freezer for several months, allowing you to enjoy homemade energy bars whenever hunger strikes.

Benefits of Homemade Energy Bars

Homemade energy bars offer numerous benefits compared to their store-bought counterparts. Not only are they free from artificial additives, preservatives, and refined sugars, but they also allow you to control the quality and quantity of ingredients, ensuring that you're fueling your body with wholesome, nutrient-dense foods.

Additionally, making energy bars at home can be a cost-effective alternative to purchasing pre-packaged bars, as you can buy ingredients in bulk and customize the recipe to suit your budget. Plus, by preparing your snacks in advance, you can save time and avoid the temptation of reaching for less healthy options when hunger strikes.

Conclusion

In conclusion, homemade energy bars are a delicious, nutritious, and convenient snack option that's perfect for busy individuals on the go. By making energy bars at home, you can enjoy the benefits of wholesome ingredients, customizable recipes, and cost-effective snacking solutions that support your health and well-being. Whether you're looking for a quick breakfast option, a pre-workout snack, or a mid-afternoon pick-me-up, homemade energy bars are sure to satisfy your cravings and keep you fueled throughout the day. Get creative in the kitchen, experiment with different flavor combinations, and discover the joy of making your own delicious and nutritious energy bars at home.

Conclusion

As we wrap up Chapter 5: Snack Time Solutions, we hope you've discovered a variety of delicious and nutritious snack options to incorporate into your daily routine. Snacking doesn't have to be complicated or unhealthy—in fact, with the right ingredients and recipes, it can be a delightful way to support your health and well-being. By choosing wholesome snacks made with real, nutrient-dense ingredients, you can fuel your body with the energy it needs to power through your day and feel your best. Whether you're enjoying a handful of nutritious trail mix, dipping crunchy veggie sticks into creamy hummus, or indulging in a homemade energy bar, remember that every snack is an opportunity to nourish your body and treat yourself well. We encourage you to get creative in the kitchen, experiment with different flavors and ingredients, and find the snack combinations that work best for you. With a little planning and preparation, you can enjoy delicious and satisfying snacks that support your health goals and keep you feeling energized and satisfied all day long. Here's to happy snacking and a healthier, happier you!

Chapter 6

"Desserts for Diabetics"

**Introduction **

Indulging in desserts is often considered a luxury, but for individuals with diabetes, it can sometimes feel like a forbidden pleasure. However, with the right knowledge and approach, enjoying delicious desserts can be a part of a balanced diabetic diet. Chapter 6: Desserts for Diabetics explores creative and satisfying ways to satisfy your sweet tooth while managing blood sugar levels effectively. In this chapter, we delve into various dessert options specially crafted for individuals with diabetes. From sugar-free baking basics to fruit-based sweets and guilt-free chocolate treats, these recipes are designed to deliver on flavor without compromising on health. By emphasizing nutrient-dense ingredients, mindful portion control, and smart cooking techniques, these desserts offer a delightful way to indulge responsibly. We understand the importance of desserts in bringing joy and satisfaction to everyday life. With our collection of diabetic-friendly dessert recipes, you can embrace the pleasure of sweet treats while supporting your overall health and well-being. Whether you're craving a decadent chocolate brownie, a refreshing fruit sorbet, or a creamy cheesecake, there's a dessert option to suit every taste and occasion. Join us on a journey through the world of diabetic-friendly desserts, where flavor meets functionality, and indulgence meets balance. Let's explore the art of creating desserts that nourish the body, delight the senses, and bring sweetness to life, one delicious bite at a time.

6.1. Sugar-Free Baking Basics

In the realm of desserts for diabetics, mastering the art of sugar-free baking is a game-changer. Sugar is a staple ingredient in traditional baking, providing sweetness, moisture, and texture to a wide range of treats. However, for individuals managing diabetes, excessive sugar consumption can lead to spikes in blood sugar levels, making it crucial to find alternative ways to achieve sweetness without compromising on flavor or texture.

Understanding Sugar Substitutes

When it comes to sugar-free baking, the first step is to familiarize yourself with various sugar substitutes available on the market. These substitutes come in different forms, including natural sweeteners like stevia, monk fruit extract, erythritol, and xylitol, as well as artificial sweeteners such as aspartame, sucralose, and saccharin. Each sweetener has its own unique taste profile, sweetness level, and baking properties, so it's essential to experiment and find the ones that work best for your recipes and personal preferences.

Balancing Sweetness and Flavor

In sugar-free baking, achieving the right balance of sweetness and flavor is key to creating delicious treats that satisfy your cravings without sending your blood sugar levels on a rollercoaster ride. Since sugar substitutes vary in sweetness intensity, it may take some trial and error to determine the ideal amount for your recipes. Start by using small amounts of sweetener and gradually adjust to taste, keeping in mind that some sweeteners can have a slightly different aftertaste compared to sugar.

Enhancing Texture and Moisture

In addition to sweetness, sugar also plays a crucial role in providing moisture and texture to baked goods. Without sugar, desserts can sometimes turn out dry, dense, or crumbly. To overcome this challenge, sugar-free bakers often rely on alternative ingredients and techniques to achieve the desired texture and moisture level in their treats. For example, using ingredients like applesauce, mashed bananas, Greek yogurt, or nut butter can add moisture and richness to baked goods without the need for added sugar. Additionally, incorporating ingredients like almond flour, coconut flour, or oat fiber can help improve the texture and structure of sugar-free desserts.

Embracing Flavorful Additions

While sugar-free baking may require some adjustments, it also presents an opportunity to get creative with flavor. By incorporating ingredients like spices, extracts, citrus zest, and nuts into your recipes, you can enhance the flavor profile of your desserts and create unique, delicious treats that are anything but boring. Experiment with different flavor combinations and ingredients to discover new and exciting ways to enjoy sugar-free baking.

Conclusion

In conclusion, mastering the art of sugar-free baking opens up a world of possibilities for individuals managing diabetes who want to enjoy delicious desserts without compromising their health. By understanding the various sugar substitutes available, balancing sweetness and flavor, enhancing texture and moisture, and embracing flavorful additions, you can create a wide range of sugar-free treats that are both satisfying and satisfying. With a little creativity and experimentation, you can indulge your sweet tooth while keeping your blood sugar levels in check, proving that sugar-free baking can be both delicious and nutritious.

6.2. Fruit-Based Sweets

In the realm of desserts for diabetics, fruit-based sweets offer a delightful combination of natural sweetness, vibrant flavors, and nutritional benefits. Fruits are not only rich in vitamins, minerals, and antioxidants but also contain natural sugars, making them a perfect ingredient for creating delicious desserts without the need for added sugars. From simple fruit salads to elegant fruit tarts, there are countless ways to incorporate fruits into your sweet treats while keeping your blood sugar levels in check.

Harnessing the Natural Sweetness of Fruits

One of the most appealing aspects of fruit-based sweets is the natural sweetness inherent in fruits themselves. Fruits like berries, apples, oranges, and mangoes contain natural sugars such as fructose, which provides sweetness without causing rapid spikes in blood sugar levels. By harnessing the natural sweetness of fruits, you can create desserts that are satisfyingly sweet without the need for added sugars or artificial sweeteners.

Exploring Flavor Combinations

In addition to sweetness, fruits offer a wide range of flavors, from tangy and tart to sweet and tropical. Experimenting with different fruit combinations allows you to create desserts that tantalize your taste buds and satisfy your cravings. For example, pairing sweet strawberries with tangy kiwi or combining juicy peaches with creamy yogurt can create a symphony of flavors that elevate your fruit-based desserts to new heights.

Creative Dessert Ideas

When it comes to fruit-based sweets, the possibilities are endless. Whether you're craving a refreshing summer treat or a cozy winter indulgence, there's a fruit-based dessert to suit every occasion. Here are just a few creative ideas to inspire your culinary adventures:

1. Fruit Salad with Mint-Lime Dressing: Combine a variety of fresh fruits such as watermelon, pineapple, grapes, and mint leaves in a large bowl. Drizzle with a refreshing dressing made from lime juice, honey, and fresh mint for a burst of flavor.

2. Grilled Fruit Skewers: Thread chunks of pineapple, mango, and banana onto skewers and grill until caramelized. Serve with a dollop of Greek yogurt and a sprinkle of cinnamon for a delicious and nutritious dessert.

3. Berry Crumble: Toss mixed berries with a splash of lemon juice and a sprinkle of stevia or erythritol. Top with a crumble made from oats, almond flour, and coconut oil, and bake until golden brown and bubbly.

4. Frozen Fruit Popsicles: Blend your favorite fruits with coconut water or Greek yogurt and pour into popsicle molds. Freeze until solid for a refreshing and healthy treat on hot summer days.

Conclusion

In conclusion, fruit-based sweets offer a delectable way to satisfy your sweet tooth while staying mindful of your blood sugar levels. By harnessing the natural sweetness and vibrant flavors of fruits, you can create desserts that are not only delicious but also nutritious and satisfying. Whether you prefer simple fruit salads, elegant fruit tarts, or creative fruit-based creations, there's a dessert to suit every taste and occasion. So embrace the natural goodness of fruits and indulge in guilt-free sweetness that nourishes both body and soul.

6.3. Guilt-Free Chocolate Treats

Indulging in chocolate treats is a pleasure that many people with diabetes may feel they need to forgo due to concerns about blood sugar spikes. However, with the right approach, it's possible to enjoy delicious chocolate desserts without guilt or worry. By incorporating high-quality ingredients, mindful portion control, and smart preparation techniques, you can create a variety of guilt-free chocolate treats that satisfy your cravings while supporting your health goals.

Choosing the Right Chocolate

When it comes to making guilt-free chocolate treats, the type of chocolate you use matters. Opt for high-quality dark chocolate with a cocoa content of at least 70% or higher. Dark chocolate contains less sugar than milk chocolate and is rich in antioxidants, which may have benefits for heart health and blood sugar control. Additionally, choosing sugar-free or stevia-sweetened chocolate can further reduce the sugar content of your desserts without sacrificing flavor.

Mindful Portion Control

While chocolate can be part of a balanced diet for individuals with diabetes, portion control is key. Instead of indulging in large servings of chocolate treats, savor small portions mindfully. Enjoying a square or two of dark chocolate after a meal can satisfy your sweet tooth without causing significant spikes in blood sugar levels. Pairing chocolate with protein-rich foods such as nuts or Greek yogurt can also help mitigate its impact on blood sugar.

Smart Ingredient Swaps

When making guilt-free chocolate treats, consider using healthier alternatives to traditional ingredients to reduce the overall sugar and carbohydrate content of your desserts. For example, you can substitute refined sugars with natural sweeteners like stevia, erythritol, or monk fruit extract. Additionally, using almond flour or coconut flour instead of white flour can lower the glycemic index of your treats while adding a nutty flavor and a boost of fiber.

Creative Chocolate Dessert Ideas

From rich and decadent brownies to creamy and velvety mousses, there are countless ways to incorporate chocolate into guilt-free desserts for diabetics. Here are some creative ideas to inspire your chocolate creations:

1. Avocado Chocolate Mousse: Blend ripe avocados with unsweetened cocoa powder, vanilla extract, and a natural sweetener of your choice until smooth and creamy. Serve chilled for a luscious and nutrient-rich dessert.

2. Chocolate-Covered Strawberries: Dip fresh strawberries in melted dark chocolate and allow them to set on a parchment-lined baking sheet. Enjoy as a simple yet elegant treat that satisfies your chocolate cravings and provides a dose of antioxidants.

3. Flourless Chocolate Cake: Make a decadent flourless chocolate cake using almond flour, cocoa powder, eggs, and a sugar-free sweetener.

Serve with a dollop of whipped cream or a sprinkle of chopped nuts for added indulgence.

4. Chocolate-Coconut Energy Bites: Mix together shredded coconut, almond flour, cocoa powder, almond butter, and a natural sweetener to form a dough. Roll into bite-sized balls and refrigerate until firm for a convenient and satisfying snack.

Conclusion

In conclusion, enjoying chocolate treats as part of a balanced diet for individuals with diabetes is not only possible but also deliciously satisfying. By choosing high-quality dark chocolate, practicing mindful portion control, and making smart ingredient swaps, you can indulge in guilt-free chocolate desserts that support your health and well-being. Whether you prefer rich and fudgy brownies, creamy chocolate mousse, or simple chocolate-covered fruits, there's a guilt-free chocolate treat to suit every taste and occasion. So embrace the pleasure of chocolate in moderation and delight in the sweet moments it brings to your life.

Conclusion to Chapter 6: Desserts for Diabetics

In conclusion, Chapter 6: Desserts for Diabetics serves as a testament to the idea that individuals with diabetes can enjoy delicious desserts without compromising their health goals. Through innovative recipes and mindful approaches to ingredient selection and preparation, we've demonstrated that dessert time can be both pleasurable and nutritious. By incorporating sugar-free baking basics, fruit-based sweets, and guilt-free chocolate treats into your culinary repertoire, you can expand your dessert options while managing your blood sugar levels effectively. With an emphasis on whole, nutrient-dense ingredients and portion control, these desserts offer a satisfying way to indulge responsibly. As you explore the recipes and techniques outlined in this chapter, we encourage you to get creative in the kitchen and tailor the desserts to your taste preferences and dietary needs. With a little experimentation and a lot of passion, you can discover new favorites and enjoy the sweet moments that life has to offer, all while supporting your journey towards optimal health and well-being.

Chapter 7

"Beverages for Blood Sugar Control"

Introduction:

Welcome to the comprehensive guide on beverages for blood sugar control. In this chapter, we explore a variety of refreshing and nutritious drink options designed to help individuals manage their blood sugar levels effectively while enjoying delicious flavors and staying hydrated. With an emphasis on low-glycemic index ingredients and mindful beverage choices, this chapter aims to empower readers with the knowledge and inspiration needed to make healthier drink choices that support overall health and well-being. As we delve into the world of beverages for blood sugar control, we'll discover the benefits of incorporating low-glycemic index beverages into your daily routine, explore creative recipes and flavor combinations, and learn how to make informed choices that promote stable blood sugar levels and optimal hydration. Whether you're seeking refreshing smoothies, herbal teas, or guilt-free lemonades, this chapter has something for everyone looking to maintain balanced blood sugar levels without sacrificing taste or enjoyment. Join us on a journey through a variety of flavorful and nourishing beverages that prioritize health and wellness while satisfying your taste buds and quenching your thirst. Let's raise a glass to better blood sugar control and vibrant well-being!

7.1 Herbal Teas and Infusions

Herbal teas and infusions offer a refreshing and flavorful way to stay hydrated while providing potential health benefits, including aiding in blood sugar control. Unlike traditional teas derived from the Camellia sinensis plant, herbal teas are made from various herbs, spices, flowers, and fruits, each with its unique taste profile and potential medicinal properties. In this section, we explore the world of herbal teas and infusions, highlighting their role in promoting hydration and supporting blood sugar management.

Understanding Herbal Teas and Infusions

Herbal teas, also known as tisanes, have been consumed for centuries for their medicinal properties and soothing effects. Unlike black, green, or white teas, which come from the Camellia sinensis plant, herbal teas are made by steeping various plant materials, such as leaves, flowers, roots, and seeds, in hot water. This infusion process extracts the flavors, aromas, and beneficial compounds from the plant materials, creating a flavorful and aromatic beverage.

Health Benefits of Herbal Teas

Many herbs and botanicals used in herbal teas are renowned for their potential health benefits, including blood sugar regulation. For example, cinnamon tea, made from cinnamon bark, has been shown to improve insulin sensitivity and lower blood sugar levels in some studies. Similarly, ginger tea may help lower fasting blood sugar levels and improve insulin sensitivity in people with type 2 diabetes. Other herbs commonly used in herbal teas, such as chamomile, peppermint, and hibiscus, may also have beneficial effects on blood sugar control. Chamomile tea, known for its calming properties, may help lower blood sugar levels and reduce insulin resistance. Peppermint tea, with its refreshing flavor, may aid in digestion and potentially support blood sugar management. Hibiscus tea is rich in antioxidants and may help lower blood pressure and improve cholesterol levels, which are important factors in overall diabetes management.

How to Incorporate Herbal Teas into Your Routine

Incorporating herbal teas and infusions into your daily routine is simple and enjoyable. Start by exploring different herbal blends and flavors to find ones that appeal to your taste preferences. Experiment with brewing techniques, such as steeping times and water temperatures, to achieve the desired strength and flavor intensity.

Consider enjoying herbal teas as part of your morning ritual, afternoon pick-me-up, or evening wind-down routine. They can be enjoyed hot or cold, depending on your preference and the season. To enhance the flavor and health benefits of herbal teas, consider adding natural sweeteners like stevia or a touch of citrus for brightness.

Conclusion: Embracing the Benefits of Herbal Teas

In conclusion, herbal teas and infusions offer a delicious and healthful way to support blood sugar control and overall well-being. By incorporating a variety of herbs and botanicals into your beverage rotation, you can enjoy a diverse array of flavors while potentially reaping the benefits of their medicinal properties. Whether you prefer the soothing warmth of chamomile, the invigorating zest of ginger, or the floral notes of hibiscus, there's a herbal tea to suit every taste and occasion. Embrace the ritual of brewing and savoring herbal teas as part of your daily routine, and experience the joy of nourishing your body and soul with every sip.

7.2 Refreshing Sugar-Free Lemonades

Lemonade, with its tangy flavor and refreshing qualities, is a beloved beverage enjoyed by many. However, traditional lemonades are often loaded with sugar, making them unsuitable for individuals managing their blood sugar levels. In this section, we explore the world of sugar-free lemonades, offering delicious alternatives that quench your thirst without causing spikes in blood sugar.

The Appeal of Sugar-Free Lemonades

Sugar-free lemonades offer a guilt-free way to enjoy the classic taste of lemonade without the negative impact on blood sugar levels. By using natural sweeteners or sugar substitutes, such as stevia, erythritol, or monk fruit extract, these lemonades deliver the perfect balance of sweetness and tartness without the need for added sugars. As a result, they provide a refreshing and hydrating option for individuals looking to manage their blood sugar levels while staying hydrated.

Varieties of Sugar-Free Lemonades

There are numerous variations of sugar-free lemonades to suit every taste preference and occasion. From classic lemonade made with fresh lemon juice to creatively flavored options infused with herbs, fruits, or spices, the possibilities are endless. Some popular variations include:

1. **Classic Sugar-Free Lemonade**: Made with freshly squeezed lemon juice, water, and a sugar substitute, classic sugar-free lemonade offers a simple yet satisfying way to quench your thirst.

2. **Berry Lemonade**: Combining the tartness of lemons with the sweetness of berries, berry lemonade is a delightful twist on the traditional recipe. Common berries used include strawberries, raspberries, blueberries, or blackberries, adding both flavor and antioxidants.

3. **Minty Lemonade**: Infused with fresh mint leaves, minty lemonade offers a refreshing and invigorating flavor profile. The coolness of the mint complements the tanginess of the lemons, creating a harmonious blend of flavors.

4. **Spicy Lemonade**: For those who enjoy a bit of heat, spicy lemonade incorporates ingredients like cayenne pepper or ginger for an added kick. The spiciness adds depth to the flavor profile, making it a unique and memorable beverage option.

Tips for Making Sugar-Free Lemonades

Creating delicious sugar-free lemonades at home is simple and fun. Start by selecting ripe, juicy lemons and squeezing them to extract their flavorful juice. Experiment with different sweeteners and flavorings to find combinations that suit your taste preferences. Consider adding fresh herbs, such as basil, rosemary, or thyme, for added complexity and aroma. To enhance the visual appeal of your lemonades, garnish each glass with a slice of lemon or a sprig of mint.

Conclusion: Enjoying Sugar-Free Lemonades for Blood Sugar Control

In conclusion, sugar-free lemonades offer a delightful and hydrating beverage option for individuals seeking to manage their blood sugar levels. With their tangy flavor, refreshing qualities, and versatility, sugar-free lemonades can be enjoyed on their own or paired with meals and snacks. By exploring different variations and experimenting with ingredients, you can create custom lemonade recipes that suit your taste preferences and dietary needs. Whether you prefer classic lemonade, fruity infusions, or bold flavor combinations, there's a sugar-free lemonade recipe to satisfy every palate. Embrace the joy of sipping on a cool, refreshing glass of lemonade without worrying about its impact on your blood sugar levels.

7.3 Low-Glycemic Index Smoothies

In the realm of beverages for blood sugar control, low-glycemic index smoothies emerge as a versatile and satisfying option. These nutritious concoctions not only offer a delicious way to stay hydrated but also provide a convenient means to incorporate essential nutrients into one's diet without causing spikes in blood sugar levels. In this section, we delve into the world of low-glycemic index smoothies, exploring their benefits, ingredients, and creative recipes.

Understanding the Glycemic Index

Before delving into low-glycemic index smoothies, it's essential to understand the concept of the glycemic index (GI). The GI measures how quickly carbohydrates in a particular food raise blood sugar levels. Foods with a high GI cause rapid spikes in blood sugar, while those with a low GI are digested more slowly, resulting in gradual increases in blood sugar levels. Low-GI foods are often preferred by individuals seeking to manage their blood sugar levels effectively.

Benefits of Low-Glycemic Index Smoothies

Low-glycemic index smoothies offer several benefits for individuals looking to control their blood sugar levels while enjoying delicious and nutrient-rich beverages:

1. **Stable Blood Sugar Levels**: By incorporating ingredients with a low GI, such as leafy greens, berries, and non-starchy vegetables, low-glycemic index smoothies help stabilize blood sugar levels, reducing the risk of sudden spikes and crashes.

2. **Sustained Energy**: Unlike high-GI foods that provide a quick energy boost followed by a crash, low-glycemic index smoothies

provide sustained energy throughout the day, promoting feelings of satiety and preventing hunger cravings.

3. **Nutrient Density**: Low-glycemic index smoothies are packed with essential nutrients, including vitamins, minerals, fiber, and antioxidants, derived from fruits, vegetables, nuts, seeds, and other wholesome ingredients. These nutrients support overall health and well-being while contributing to optimal blood sugar management.

4. **Weight Management**: Incorporating low-glycemic index smoothies into a balanced diet can support weight management goals by promoting feelings of fullness and reducing calorie intake from high-GI snacks and beverages.

Ingredients for Low-Glycemic Index Smoothies

Creating delicious and nutritious low-glycemic index smoothies is simple and customizable. Start with a liquid base such as water, unsweetened almond milk, coconut water, or herbal tea. Then, add low-GI fruits like berries, cherries, apples, pears, and citrus fruits. Incorporate leafy greens such as spinach, kale, or Swiss chard for added fiber and nutrients. Enhance the flavor and nutritional profile with healthy fats from ingredients like avocado, chia seeds, flaxseeds, or nut butter. Finally, add protein sources such as Greek yogurt, silken tofu, or protein powder to promote satiety and muscle recovery.

Creative Low-Glycemic Index Smoothie Recipes

Here are a few creative low-glycemic index smoothie recipes to inspire your culinary adventures:

1. **Berry Green Smoothie**: Blend together spinach, mixed berries, avocado, Greek yogurt, and a splash of coconut water for a refreshing and nutrient-packed beverage.

2. **Tropical Paradise Smoothie**: Combine pineapple, mango, banana, coconut milk, and a handful of spinach for a taste of the tropics without the blood sugar spike.

3. **Chocolate Peanut Butter Smoothie**: Blend unsweetened cocoa powder, banana, peanut butter, spinach, and almond milk for a decadent yet nutritious treat that satisfies cravings without compromising blood sugar control.

Conclusion: Embracing Low-Glycemic Index Smoothies for Blood Sugar Control

In conclusion, low-glycemic index smoothies offer a delicious, convenient, and nutritious way to support blood sugar management goals. By incorporating ingredients with a low GI, these beverages provide sustained energy, promote satiety, and deliver essential nutrients without causing spikes in blood sugar levels. With endless flavor combinations and creative recipes to explore, low-glycemic index smoothies empower individuals to enjoy flavorful beverages while prioritizing their health and well-being. Whether enjoyed as a meal replacement, post-workout snack, or refreshing treat, low-GI smoothies are a valuable addition to any balanced diet focused on blood sugar control.

Conclusion:

In conclusion, beverages play a crucial role in maintaining stable blood sugar levels and supporting overall health and wellness. Throughout this chapter, we've explored a diverse array of options, from herbal teas and infused waters to refreshing lemonades and nutrient-packed smoothies, all designed to help individuals manage their blood sugar effectively while enjoying delicious flavors and staying hydrated.

By prioritizing low-glycemic index ingredients, mindful beverage choices, and creative recipes, individuals can take control of their blood sugar levels and make positive strides towards better health outcomes. Whether enjoyed as a standalone refreshment, a post-workout recovery drink, or a complement to a balanced meal, these beverages offer a satisfying and nutritious way to support blood sugar control and overall well-being. As you embark on your journey to better blood sugar management, remember to listen to your body, experiment with different flavors and ingredients, and find what works best for you. With the knowledge and inspiration gained from this chapter, you have the tools to make informed beverage choices that nourish your body, satisfy your taste buds, and support your journey towards a healthier, happier life. Cheers to your health and vitality!

Chapter 8

"Eating Out with Diabetes"

Introduction

Eating out can be a source of enjoyment and social connection, but for individuals managing diabetes, it also presents unique challenges. Making healthy choices while dining out is crucial for maintaining stable blood sugar levels and overall well-being. In this chapter, we will explore strategies and tips for eating out with diabetes, empowering individuals to make informed choices and enjoy dining experiences without compromising their health. Navigating restaurant menus can be daunting, with tempting dishes often high in carbohydrates, sugars, and unhealthy fats. However, armed with knowledge and planning, individuals with diabetes can confidently navigate restaurant meals while making choices that align with their dietary needs and health goals. From selecting appropriate menu items to managing portion sizes and handling social situations, this chapter will provide practical guidance for eating out with diabetes. We'll delve into topics such as making smart menu choices, controlling portion sizes, and developing effective dining strategies for social gatherings. By equipping readers with the tools and strategies needed to make healthier choices, this chapter aims to empower individuals with diabetes to dine out with confidence, enjoy delicious meals, and maintain optimal blood sugar control.

8.1. Making Smart Menu Choices

Making smart menu choices is essential for individuals managing diabetes when dining out. With careful consideration and awareness, it's possible to enjoy restaurant meals while keeping blood sugar levels in check and supporting overall health. In this section, we'll explore strategies and tips for making informed decisions when selecting dishes from restaurant menus, ensuring a satisfying and diabetes-friendly dining experience.

Understanding Nutritional Information:

One of the first steps in making smart menu choices is understanding the nutritional information provided by restaurants. Many establishments now offer detailed information about the calorie, carbohydrate, fat, and protein content of their dishes. Taking the time to review this information can help individuals make choices that align with their dietary needs and blood sugar management goals.

Focus on Whole Foods:

When browsing the menu, prioritize dishes that feature whole, minimally processed ingredients. Opt for lean proteins such as grilled chicken or fish, and choose side dishes that include plenty of vegetables and whole grains. These nutrient-dense options provide essential vitamins, minerals, and fiber while minimizing added sugars and unhealthy fats.

Watch Portion Sizes:

Portion control is key when dining out with diabetes. Many restaurant servings are larger than necessary, leading to overeating and potential spikes in blood sugar levels. Consider sharing an entrée with a dining companion or asking for a half portion to help control portion sizes and avoid overindulgence.

Be Mindful of Hidden Sugars:

Beware of hidden sugars lurking in restaurant dishes, especially in sauces, dressings, and marinades. Opt for dishes that are prepared with minimal added sugars, and ask for sauces and dressings on the side so you can control the amount you consume. Choosing grilled, steamed, or baked options over fried or breaded dishes can also help reduce added sugars in your meal.

Customize Your Order:

Don't hesitate to customize your order to suit your dietary needs and preferences. Most restaurants are willing to accommodate special requests, such as substituting steamed vegetables for French fries or requesting grilled instead of breaded chicken. By advocating for yourself and communicating your needs clearly, you can create a meal that supports your blood sugar management goals.

Stay Hydrated:

Remember to stay hydrated while dining out by drinking water or other unsweetened beverages. Limiting sugary sodas, sweetened teas, and alcoholic beverages can help prevent unnecessary spikes in blood sugar levels and promote overall hydration and well-being.

Conclusion:

Making smart menu choices is a vital aspect of dining out with diabetes. By understanding nutritional information, focusing on whole foods, watching portion sizes, being mindful of hidden sugars, customizing your order, and staying hydrated, individuals can enjoy delicious restaurant meals while supporting their blood sugar management goals and overall health. With practice and awareness, dining out can be a satisfying and enjoyable experience that contributes to a healthy lifestyle for individuals living with diabetes.

8.2. Portion Control Tips

Portion control is a crucial aspect of managing diabetes, especially when dining out. Controlling portion sizes helps regulate blood sugar levels and promotes weight management, both of which are essential for overall health. In this section, we'll explore effective portion control tips that individuals with diabetes can employ when eating out, empowering them to make healthier choices and maintain optimal blood sugar control.

1. Use Visual Cues:

Visual cues can help individuals estimate appropriate portion sizes when dining out. For example, a serving of protein should be about the size of a deck of cards, while a serving of carbohydrates, such as rice or pasta, should be approximately the size of a tennis ball. By mentally comparing the portions served to these visual references, individuals can better control their intake.

2. Share Entrées:

Many restaurant portions are oversized, containing more food than necessary for one person. To avoid overeating, consider sharing an entrée with a dining companion. Sharing not only helps control portion sizes but also reduces costs and minimizes food waste, making it a win-win situation for both health and sustainability.

3. Start with a Salad:

Starting your meal with a salad or a broth-based soup can help fill you up with low-calorie, nutrient-rich foods before the main course arrives. This can help curb your appetite and prevent overeating when the main dish is served. Opt for salads with plenty of vegetables and lean protein, and dress them with vinaigrette or other low-calorie dressings.

4. Request Half Portions:

Don't hesitate to ask your server if the restaurant offers half portions or the option to customize your meal size. Many establishments are willing to accommodate special requests to meet the needs of their patrons. Ordering a half portion can help prevent the temptation to overeat while still allowing you to enjoy a variety of dishes.

5. Box Half Your Meal:

If portion sizes are generous, consider boxing up half of your meal before you start eating. This prevents mindless eating and allows you to enjoy the remainder of your meal as a leftover the next day. Not only does this strategy help control portion sizes, but it also stretches your dining budget and reduces food waste.

6. Be Mindful of Buffets:

Buffet-style dining can pose challenges for portion control, as the abundance of options can lead to overeating. To navigate buffet situations successfully, scan the offerings before filling your plate, prioritize healthier options like salads, grilled proteins, and vegetables, and use small plates to control portion sizes.

Conclusion:

Portion control is essential for individuals with diabetes to manage blood sugar levels and maintain a healthy weight. By using visual cues, sharing entrees, starting with a salad, requesting half portions, boxing half your meal, and being mindful of buffets, individuals can navigate dining out with diabetes successfully. These tips empower individuals to make informed choices, enjoy delicious meals, and support their overall health and well-being.

8.3. Dining Strategies for Social Gatherings

Social gatherings often revolve around food, presenting unique challenges for individuals with diabetes who need to carefully manage their blood sugar levels. However, with the right strategies and mindset, it's possible to navigate these situations successfully while still enjoying the company of friends and family. In this section, we'll explore effective dining strategies for social gatherings that empower individuals with diabetes to make healthier choices without feeling deprived or isolated.

Navigating Buffet-Style Events:

Buffet-style events can be particularly challenging for individuals with diabetes due to the abundance of food choices and the temptation to overeat. To navigate buffet-style events successfully, it's essential to approach them with a plan. Start by scanning all the available options before filling your plate, focusing on healthier choices like grilled proteins, salads, and vegetables. Use smaller plates to control portion sizes and avoid going back for seconds unless you're truly hungry. Remember to prioritize foods that are lower in carbohydrates and added sugars to help manage blood sugar levels.

Communicating with Hosts:

When attending social gatherings, it's helpful to communicate with the hosts ahead of time about your dietary needs. Politely explain that you have diabetes and may need to make specific food choices to manage your condition. Offer to bring a dish to share that aligns with your dietary requirements, ensuring that there will be at least one option you can enjoy guilt-free. Most hosts will appreciate your proactive approach and accommodate your needs to the best of their ability.

Being Selective with Alcoholic Beverages:

Alcoholic beverages are often served at social gatherings, but they can have a significant impact on blood sugar levels, especially if consumed in excess or mixed with sugary mixers. When choosing alcoholic beverages, opt for light beer, dry wine, or spirits mixed with sugar-free mixers or soda water. Avoid sugary cocktails, sweet wines, and flavored alcoholic beverages, which can cause blood sugar spikes. Remember to drink in moderation and alternate alcoholic beverages with water to stay hydrated and prevent overindulgence.

Mindful Eating Practices:

Practice mindful eating during social gatherings by paying attention to hunger and fullness cues, eating slowly, and savoring each bite. Take the time to engage in conversation with friends and family between bites, allowing yourself to enjoy the social aspect of the event rather than focusing solely on food. By being present and mindful during meals, you'll be less likely to overeat and more in tune with your body's signals of hunger and satiety.

Conclusion:

Social gatherings can present challenges for individuals with diabetes, but with the right strategies and mindset, it's possible to navigate these situations successfully while still enjoying delicious food and the company of loved ones. By implementing strategies such as navigating buffet-style events with a plan, communicating with hosts about dietary needs, being selective with alcoholic beverages, and practicing mindful eating, individuals with diabetes can make healthier choices and maintain optimal blood sugar control, ensuring that social gatherings remain enjoyable and fulfilling experiences.

Conclusion

In conclusion, dining out with diabetes doesn't have to be a daunting task. With careful planning, mindful choices, and effective strategies, individuals can enjoy dining experiences while successfully managing their blood sugar levels. By making smart menu choices, controlling portion sizes, and communicating with restaurant staff about dietary needs, individuals with diabetes can navigate restaurant meals with confidence and ease.

Furthermore, adopting mindful eating practices and incorporating healthy habits into dining experiences can enhance overall well-being and support long-term health goals. Remembering to prioritize nutrient-dense foods, stay hydrated, and savor each bite can contribute to a more enjoyable and satisfying dining experience.

Ultimately, eating out with diabetes is about balance, flexibility, and empowerment. By arming themselves with knowledge and implementing practical strategies, individuals can confidently navigate restaurant meals, enjoy delicious food, and maintain optimal blood sugar control, ensuring that dining out remains a pleasurable and fulfilling aspect of life.

Chapter 9

"Meal Planning and Prep"

Introduction:

In the journey of managing diabetes, meal planning and preparation play a crucial role in achieving optimal health and well-being. This chapter delves into the art of meal planning and prep, offering valuable insights and practical strategies to empower individuals with diabetes to make informed dietary choices and maintain stable blood sugar levels.

Meal planning involves thoughtful consideration of food choices, portion sizes, and timing of meals to help individuals achieve their health goals while effectively managing their blood sugar levels. By carefully selecting nutrient-dense foods and balancing macronutrients, individuals can create satisfying and nourishing meals that support overall health and diabetes management.

Through this chapter, readers will gain a deeper understanding of the principles of meal planning and prep, along with actionable tips and strategies to streamline the process and make it more manageable. From building balanced plates to utilizing weekly menu templates and embracing batch cooking techniques, individuals will discover practical tools to simplify meal preparation and set themselves up for success in their diabetes management journey.

With a focus on accessibility, flexibility, and sustainability, the strategies outlined in this chapter are designed to empower individuals to take control of their dietary choices and navigate various eating environments with confidence and ease. By incorporating these principles into their daily routine, individuals can enjoy delicious, nutritious meals that promote overall health and well-being while effectively managing their diabetes.

9.1 Building Balanced Plates

Building balanced plates is a fundamental aspect of meal planning for individuals managing diabetes. By creating meals that are well-balanced in macronutrients and rich in essential nutrients, individuals can better control their blood sugar levels and support overall health. In this section, we will explore the principles of building balanced plates, focusing on the importance of incorporating a variety of foods to create meals that are both nutritious and satisfying.

Understanding Macronutrients:

When building balanced plates, it's essential to consider the three main macronutrients: carbohydrates, protein, and fats. Carbohydrates have the most significant impact on blood sugar levels, so it's crucial to choose high-fiber, complex carbohydrates that are digested more slowly, leading to gradual rises in blood sugar levels. Good sources of complex carbohydrates include whole grains, legumes, vegetables, and fruits. Protein is essential for maintaining muscle mass, promoting satiety, and stabilizing blood sugar levels. Incorporating lean protein sources such as poultry, fish, tofu, legumes, and low-fat dairy products into meals can help balance blood sugar levels and keep hunger at bay. Healthy fats play a crucial role in heart health and satiety. Opt for sources of unsaturated fats such as avocados, nuts, seeds, and olive oil to add flavor and richness to meals without significantly affecting blood sugar levels.

Creating Balanced Meals:

A balanced plate should consist of approximately half non-starchy vegetables, one-quarter lean protein, and one-quarter whole grains or starchy vegetables. Non-starchy vegetables are low in carbohydrates and calories but rich in vitamins, minerals, and fiber, making them an excellent choice for filling up without spiking blood sugar levels. Pairing protein with carbohydrates can help slow down the absorption of sugars into the bloodstream, preventing rapid spikes in blood sugar levels. Including a variety of colors, textures, and flavors in meals can make them more enjoyable and satisfying.

Portion Control:

In addition to focusing on food choices, portion control is essential for managing blood sugar levels and preventing overeating. Using smaller plates, measuring portions, and being mindful of portion sizes can help individuals avoid consuming excess calories and carbohydrates.

Conclusion:

Building balanced plates is a cornerstone of effective meal planning for individuals with diabetes. By incorporating a variety of nutrient-dense foods in appropriate portions, individuals can create meals that promote stable blood sugar levels, provide essential nutrients, and support overall health and well-being. By following the principles outlined in this section, individuals can take control of their dietary choices, enjoy delicious and satisfying meals, and better manage their diabetes.

9.2 Weekly Menu Templates

Creating weekly menu templates is an effective strategy for simplifying meal planning and ensuring balanced nutrition for individuals managing diabetes. By mapping out meals for the week ahead, individuals can save time, reduce stress, and maintain better control over their dietary choices. In this section, we will explore the benefits of using weekly menu templates and provide practical tips for designing balanced and delicious meal plans.

Benefits of Weekly Menu Templates:

Weekly menu templates offer several advantages for individuals with diabetes:

1. **Improved Organization:** Planning meals in advance allows individuals to organize their shopping lists, ensuring they have all the necessary ingredients on hand for the week ahead.

2. **Better Nutrient Balance:** With a weekly menu template, individuals can ensure they are consuming a variety of nutrient-dense foods, including lean proteins, whole grains, fruits, vegetables, and healthy fats, to support overall health and blood sugar management.

3. **Time and Cost Savings:** By planning meals in advance, individuals can streamline their grocery shopping trips, minimize food waste, and potentially save money by purchasing ingredients in bulk or taking advantage of sales and discounts.

4. **Reduced Decision-Making:** Having a predetermined meal plan for the week eliminates the need to make last-minute decisions about what to eat, reducing decision fatigue and the temptation to choose less healthy options.

Designing Weekly Menu Templates:

When designing weekly menu templates for individuals with diabetes, it's essential to consider their dietary preferences, nutritional needs, and lifestyle factors. Here are some tips for creating effective menu plans:

1. **Include Variety:** Incorporate a diverse range of foods from all food groups to ensure adequate nutrient intake and prevent boredom. Aim for a balance of different colors, flavors, and textures in each meal.

2. **Mindful Carbohydrate Choices:** Pay attention to carbohydrate portions and choose high-fiber, low-glycemic index options such as whole grains, legumes, and non-starchy vegetables to help regulate blood sugar levels.

3. **Portion Control:** Use portion control techniques to prevent overeating and promote satiety. Consider using visual cues such as the plate method or measuring utensils to ensure appropriate portion sizes.

4. **Flexibility:** Allow for flexibility within the menu plan to accommodate changes in schedule, leftovers, or spontaneous dining occasions. Incorporate versatile ingredients that can be used in multiple recipes throughout the week.

Sample Weekly Menu Template:

Here's an example of a balanced weekly menu template for individuals with diabetes:

- **Monday:**

  - Breakfast: Whole grain oatmeal with berries and almonds

  - Lunch: Grilled chicken salad with mixed greens, vegetables, and vinaigrette

  - Dinner: Baked salmon with quinoa and roasted broccoli

- **Tuesday:**

  - Breakfast: Greek yogurt parfait with granola and sliced peaches

  - Lunch: Turkey and avocado wrap with whole grain tortilla

  - Dinner: Vegetable stir-fry with tofu and brown rice

- **Wednesday:**

  - Breakfast: Spinach and feta omelet with whole wheat toast

  - Lunch: Lentil soup with side salad and whole grain roll

  - Dinner: Baked chicken breast with sweet potato and steamed green beans

- **Thursday:**

  - Breakfast: Whole grain waffles with Greek yogurt and fresh fruit

  - Lunch: Quinoa salad with black beans, corn, and avocado

  - Dinner: Turkey meatballs with marinara sauce over whole wheat pasta

- **Friday:**

  - Breakfast: Smoothie with spinach, banana, almond milk, and protein powder

  - Lunch: Grilled vegetable and hummus wrap with whole grain pita

  - Dinner: Shrimp stir-fry with vegetables and cauliflower rice

Conclusion:

Weekly menu templates are invaluable tools for individuals managing diabetes, providing structure, organization, and support for making healthy food choices. By following the principles outlined in this section and customizing menu plans to meet individual needs and preferences, individuals can simplify meal planning, improve dietary adherence, and achieve better blood sugar control. With careful planning and attention to balanced nutrition, individuals can enjoy delicious and satisfying meals while effectively managing their diabetes.

9.3 Batch Cooking for Convenience

Batch cooking is a meal preparation strategy that involves cooking large quantities of food in advance and portioning it out for future meals. This approach offers numerous benefits for individuals managing diabetes, including saving time, reducing stress, and promoting healthier eating habits. In this section, we will explore the advantages of batch cooking and provide practical tips for incorporating this method into a diabetes-friendly meal plan.

Benefits of Batch Cooking:

Batch cooking offers several advantages for individuals with diabetes:

1. **Time Savings:** By preparing multiple meals at once, individuals can significantly reduce the amount of time spent in the kitchen on a daily basis. This is especially beneficial for those with busy schedules or limited time for meal preparation.

2. **Consistent Portion Control:** Batch cooking allows for precise portioning of meals, helping individuals manage their carbohydrate intake and control their blood sugar levels more effectively.

3. **Cost Efficiency:** Buying ingredients in bulk for batch cooking can be more cost-effective than purchasing smaller quantities. Additionally, batch cooking can help reduce food waste by using ingredients efficiently and repurposing leftovers.

4. **Healthier Food Choices:** With pre-prepared meals readily available, individuals are less likely to rely on convenience foods or takeout, which are often high in calories, unhealthy fats, and added sugars. Batch cooking promotes the consumption of homemade, nutritious meals made with fresh ingredients.

Tips for Successful Batch Cooking:

To maximize the benefits of batch cooking, consider the following tips:

1. **Plan Ahead:** Before starting a batch cooking session, take some time to plan your meals for the week and create a shopping list. Choose recipes that are suitable for batch cooking and can be easily reheated or frozen.

2. **Invest in Quality Containers:** Invest in airtight containers or freezer-safe bags to store pre-prepared meals. Label containers with the date and contents to ensure freshness and easy identification.

3. **Choose Versatile Ingredients:** Select ingredients that can be used in multiple recipes to minimize waste and simplify meal preparation. For example, cook a large batch of brown rice or quinoa that can be portioned out and paired with different proteins and vegetables throughout the week.

4. **Use Time-Saving Cooking Methods:** Utilize time-saving cooking methods such as slow cooking, pressure cooking, or one-pan meals to streamline the batch cooking process. These methods require minimal hands-on time and can yield delicious, nutritious meals with minimal effort.

Sample Batch Cooking Menu:

Here's an example of a batch cooking menu for individuals with diabetes:

- **Protein:** Grill or bake a large batch of chicken breasts or tofu.

- **Grains:** Cook a large pot of brown rice, quinoa, or whole wheat pasta.

- **Vegetables:** Roast a variety of vegetables such as carrots, broccoli, and bell peppers.

- **Soups/Stews:** Prepare a hearty vegetable soup or turkey chili in a slow cooker.

- **Snacks:** Bake a batch of homemade energy bars or portion out mixed nuts and seeds for convenient grab-and-go snacks.

Conclusion:

Batch cooking is a valuable strategy for simplifying meal preparation, saving time, and promoting healthier eating habits for individuals managing diabetes. By incorporating batch cooking into their meal planning routine and following the tips outlined in this section, individuals can enjoy the convenience of having nutritious meals readily available while effectively managing their blood sugar levels. With a little planning and preparation, batch cooking can help individuals stay on track with their dietary goals and maintain better overall health and well-being.

Conclusion:

In conclusion, meal planning and preparation are essential components of a successful diabetes management plan. By adopting a proactive approach to meal planning and incorporating practical strategies such as building balanced plates, utilizing weekly menu templates, and embracing batch cooking techniques, individuals can take control of their dietary choices and maintain stable blood sugar levels. Through careful planning and thoughtful consideration of food choices, individuals can create a sustainable and enjoyable eating pattern that supports their overall health and well-being. By making informed decisions about portion sizes, carbohydrate intake, and meal timing, individuals can effectively manage their diabetes and reduce the risk of complications. As individuals embark on their journey of meal planning and preparation, it is important to remember that flexibility and adaptability are key. While having a structured plan in place can provide guidance and support, it is also important to listen to your body's cues and make adjustments as needed. By cultivating a mindful and intuitive approach to eating, individuals can foster a positive relationship with food and enjoy a balanced and fulfilling lifestyle, even in the face of diabetes.

Chapter 10

"Conclusion and Resources"

Introduction:

In the final chapter of our comprehensive guide, we delve into the conclusion and resources available to individuals managing diabetes. Throughout this journey, we have explored various aspects of diabetes management, from understanding the condition and making lifestyle changes to navigating social gatherings and accessing support. Now, as we draw this guide to a close, we reflect on the insights gained and highlight the valuable resources that can aid individuals in their ongoing journey towards better health and well-being.

Navigating the Conclusion and Resources:

In this concluding chapter, we consolidate the key takeaways from each section of our guide, emphasizing the importance of a holistic approach to diabetes management. We underscore the significance of celebrating progress, making informed choices, and accessing support networks to empower individuals in their journey towards optimal health. Additionally, we provide a comprehensive list of resources, including online communities, reputable websites, virtual events, mobile applications, and telehealth services, to equip individuals with the tools and information they need to thrive with diabetes.

10.1. Celebrating Progress

In the journey of managing diabetes, celebrating progress is a vital aspect of maintaining motivation, fostering resilience, and acknowledging the hard work and dedication put forth by individuals striving to achieve their health goals. While the path to optimal diabetes management may be challenging at times, it is essential to recognize and celebrate every milestone, no matter how small, along the way.

Acknowledging Achievements:

Celebrating progress involves acknowledging and celebrating achievements, whether it's reaching a target blood sugar level, adopting healthier eating habits, incorporating regular physical activity into one's routine, or successfully managing stress and emotions. Each achievement, no matter how minor, represents a step forward in the journey towards better health and well-being.

Importance of Positive Reinforcement:

Positive reinforcement plays a crucial role in sustaining motivation and commitment to long-term behavior change. By celebrating progress and recognizing achievements, individuals are more likely to stay motivated and continue making positive choices that support their diabetes management efforts. Whether it's rewarding oneself with a small treat, sharing achievements with loved ones, or keeping a journal to track progress, finding ways to celebrate successes can help maintain momentum and enthusiasm.

Reflecting on Personal Growth:

Celebrating progress also involves reflecting on personal growth and recognizing the resilience, determination, and perseverance demonstrated throughout the diabetes management journey. Each challenge overcome, setback navigated, and lesson learned contributes to personal growth and resilience, equipping individuals with the skills and confidence needed to overcome future obstacles.

Fostering a Positive Mindset:

Maintaining a positive mindset is essential in managing diabetes effectively. By celebrating progress and focusing on achievements rather than setbacks, individuals can cultivate a sense of optimism and empowerment that fuels continued progress and success. Embracing a growth mindset, which views challenges as opportunities for growth and learning, can help individuals navigate the ups and downs of diabetes management with resilience and grace.

Creating Meaningful Rituals:

Celebrating progress can be as simple as creating meaningful rituals or traditions that mark milestones along the diabetes management journey. Whether it's setting aside time each week to reflect on achievements, treating oneself to a special outing or activity, or celebrating with friends and family, finding ways to commemorate progress can instill a sense of pride and accomplishment. In conclusion, celebrating progress is an integral part of the diabetes management journey, providing motivation, reinforcement, and encouragement to individuals striving to achieve their health goals. By acknowledging achievements, fostering a positive mindset, and creating meaningful rituals, individuals can cultivate resilience, maintain motivation, and continue making progress towards optimal health and well-being despite the challenges posed by diabetes.

10.2. Additional Reading and Support

In the journey of managing diabetes, access to reliable information and support resources is essential for individuals seeking to enhance their knowledge, skills, and confidence in managing their condition effectively. Additional reading materials and support networks can provide valuable insights, practical tips, and emotional support to help individuals navigate the complexities of diabetes management and improve their overall well-being.

Exploring Comprehensive Guides and Books:

There are numerous comprehensive guides and books available that cover various aspects of diabetes management, including nutrition, exercise, medication management, blood sugar monitoring, and emotional well-being. These resources often provide evidence-based information, practical strategies, and real-life stories that resonate with individuals living with diabetes, empowering them to take control of their health and make informed decisions.

Delving into Research Articles and Journals:

For those seeking in-depth knowledge about specific topics related to diabetes management, research articles and journals can be valuable sources of information. These publications often present the latest findings from scientific studies, clinical trials, and medical research, offering insights into emerging trends, treatment options, and best practices in diabetes care. Accessing reputable medical journals and peer-reviewed articles can help individuals stay informed about advancements in diabetes management and treatment.

Engaging with Online Forums and Communities:

Online forums and communities provide platforms for individuals living with diabetes to connect, share experiences, ask questions, and offer support to one another. These virtual communities can be invaluable sources of encouragement, empathy, and practical advice, especially for those navigating the challenges of diabetes management. By participating in online discussions, individuals can gain insights from others facing similar challenges, find inspiration from success stories, and build meaningful connections with peers.

Attending Workshops and Support Groups:

Many organizations and healthcare providers offer workshops, seminars, and support groups specifically tailored to individuals living with diabetes. These in-person or virtual events provide opportunities for education, skill-building, and peer support in a supportive and empathetic environment. By attending these sessions, individuals can learn from experts, share experiences with others, and gain practical strategies for managing their diabetes more effectively.

Accessing Online Resources and Websites:

There are numerous websites and online resources dedicated to diabetes education, support, and advocacy. These platforms offer a wealth of information, including articles, videos, webinars, interactive tools, and downloadable resources, covering various aspects of diabetes management and self-care. By exploring these online resources, individuals can access reliable information, practical tips, and tools to support their diabetes management journey. In conclusion, additional reading materials and support resources play a crucial role in empowering individuals with diabetes to enhance their knowledge, skills, and confidence in managing their condition effectively. Whether through comprehensive guides, research articles, online forums, workshops, or online resources, accessing reliable information and support networks can help individuals navigate the complexities of diabetes management and improve their overall well-being.

10.3. Online Communities and Resources for Diabetics

Online communities and resources play a pivotal role in supporting individuals with diabetes by providing a platform for education, connection, and empowerment. These virtual spaces offer a wealth of information, peer support, and practical tools to help individuals manage their condition effectively and improve their quality of life.

Connecting with Others:

Online communities provide a safe and supportive environment for individuals with diabetes to connect with others facing similar challenges. These communities often feature discussion forums, social media groups, and virtual support networks where members can share experiences, ask questions, offer advice, and provide encouragement. By connecting with others who understand their journey, individuals with diabetes can find solace, inspiration, and a sense of belonging.

Accessing Reliable Information:

Many reputable websites and online platforms are dedicated to providing reliable information and resources for individuals with diabetes. These resources cover various aspects of diabetes management, including nutrition, exercise, medication, blood sugar monitoring, and emotional well-being. By accessing trustworthy, information from reputable sources, individuals can make informed decisions about their health and lifestyle choices.

Participating in Webinars and Virtual Events:

Webinars, virtual conferences, and online events offer opportunities for individuals with diabetes to learn from experts, participate in interactive sessions, and gain practical insights into managing their condition. These virtual gatherings cover a wide range of topics, such as diabetes management techniques, healthy living strategies, and advancements in treatment options. By participating in these events, individuals can expand their knowledge, acquire new skills, and stay up-to-date with the latest developments in diabetes care.

Utilizing Mobile Applications and Digital Tools:

Mobile applications and digital tools designed for diabetes management provide convenient and accessible resources for individuals seeking to track their health metrics, monitor their blood sugar levels, manage their medications, and make healthier lifestyle choices. These apps often feature interactive features, personalized recommendations, and user-friendly interfaces that empower individuals to take control of their health and well-being.

Accessing Support from Healthcare Professionals:

Many healthcare providers offer telehealth services and online consultations, allowing individuals with diabetes to receive personalized guidance, support, and medical advice from qualified professionals. These virtual consultations enable individuals to discuss their concerns, receive tailored recommendations, and develop personalized care plans without the need for in-person appointments. By leveraging these online resources, individuals can access timely support and guidance to optimize their diabetes management. In conclusion, online communities and resources serve as invaluable assets for individuals with diabetes, offering a wealth of information, support, and practical tools to help them navigate the complexities of managing their condition. Whether through virtual support networks, reliable websites, online events, mobile applications, or telehealth services, these online resources empower individuals to take control of their health, connect with others, and lead fulfilling lives despite their diagnosis.

Conclusion:

As we conclude our guide, we extend our gratitude to our readers for embarking on this journey with us. We recognize the challenges and complexities inherent in managing diabetes and commend the dedication and resilience of individuals striving to live well with this condition. While the road may be filled with obstacles, we have seen firsthand the power of education, empowerment, and community in overcoming them. In closing, we emphasize the importance of taking proactive steps towards self-care, seeking support when needed, and embracing the resources available to navigate the complexities of diabetes management. By harnessing the knowledge gained from this guide and leveraging the wealth of resources at their disposal, individuals with diabetes can embark on a path towards improved health, enhanced well-being, and a fulfilling life beyond their diagnosis. Together, let us celebrate progress, make informed choices, and continue to support one another in the journey towards diabetes management and beyond.